# PRAISE FOR CUR :

Lazris, a primary care geriatric physician and medical director at facilities for the frail elderly, advocates a minimalist approach to medical intervention for many chronic health problems of advanced age, including dementia. He argues that Medicare's outdated payment rules and assumptions about life expectancy are financing "an interminable search for eternal life" instead of ensuring that Medicare pays for long-term "palliative" care, ideally at home. With an insider's view, the author does an excellent job of diagnosing pervasive problems in the Medicare system. A fascinating look at how Medicare must change.
**Kirkus Reviews**

There is now a sizable choir of American physicians recruited from all corners of the profession whose voices are raised in anguish over the difficulty of practicing medicine according to their conscience. Now Dr. Lazris adds Curing Medicare to the repertoire. It is a compelling lament this is, at once, strident and compassionate. It earns Dr. Lazris a position in the front row of the choir. If only we could fill the pews.
**Nortin M Hadler MD, Author of The Last Well Person and Rethinking Aging**
**Professor of Medicine, University of North Carolina Medical School, Chapel Hill**

As a medical student, I was trained in "thorough" – the goal being to find as many problems with my patients as possible. In *Curing Medicare*, Dr. Lazris seeks to redefine "thorough" – and not simply to humanize our profession, but to protect the elderly from the harms of too much medical care. It is a passionate, but thoughtful, critique of medicine's relentless focus on numbers, unimportant measures of performance, and turning people into patients.
**H. Gilbert Welch MD, MPH, Author of Overdiagnosed: Making People Sick in the Pursuit of Health.**
**Professor of Medicine, Dartmouth Institute for Health Policy & Clinical Practice**

A trenchant analysis of the ills of the current health care regime for the elderly. Dr. Lazris's message is a timeless one: you're not sick. You're just getting older. It is not, after all, an unusual condition in the scope of human history. Throughout he warns of the perils of too much, too much surgery, too much medicine, and too high an expectation for eternal youth. It's a page turner.

**Phillip Soergel, Chairman and Professor, Department of History, University of Maryland College Park**

I recommend CURING MEDICARE for all patients, politicians, physicians, nurses and health policy thinkers. This is an important book by a very skilled individual. Somehow this man effectively transforms his frustrations with the Medicare system into wonderfully clear teaching stories and solid policy recommendations.

**Robert M Duggan, MA, Author of Breaking the Iron Triangle of Health Care Costs**

Dr. Lazris, a general internist and geriatrician, has written a wise book. All doctors in training and doctors in practice should read it, and so should their patients. Our health system has been slowly but steadily making it hard to be well. This book is well written, well researched, and makes a strong case that less is more for many of the common conditions and maladies that bring people to doctors. Organized medicine and academic medicine makes much of evidence based practice. But what happens when the evidence is weak? Read this book and judge for yourself.

**Daniel Becker, MD, MPH, Professor of Medicine, University of Virginia Medical Center**

# CURING
# MEDICARE

*One doctor's view of how our
health care system is failing the
elderly and how to fix it*

ANDY LAZRIS MD

ISBN: 1499549806
ISBN-13: 9781499549805
Library of Congress Control Number: 2014909145
CreateSpace Independent Publishing Platform
North Charleston, South Carolina

# DEDICATION

To my wonderful wife and kids, who are everything to me: Cathy, Michael, David, and Rachel. Also to my parents, Yale and Marilyn, my sister Kim and brother Mitch, as well as to Jenny, Marc, Matt, Jacob, Elana, Bryce, Theresa, Jeff, and Mia, as well as my in-laws Mary and Frank Staropoli. To my running group who had to hear all my chatter about the book for endless miles: Andres, Paula, and Mike. Finally to all those I work with, including Pat, Jill, Kathy, Erica, Michelle, Phillip, Libby, Bonnie, and all the many administrators, nurses, aides, social workers, therapists, and receptionists who have done so much to make the world I live in better. Thanks to Lou Grimmel for helping me to start my practice and continuing to inspire, to my son Michael for help with research and marketing, to my editor Christine Day who helped me finalize and improve the manuscript, and to all the primary care geriatric doctors out there taking care of their patients with love and expertise in a system that is not always very kind.

# TABLE OF CONTENTS:

# FOREWORD

# A BOOK'S JOURNEY

Several years ago I made a decision to write a book about geriatric health care delivery from the perspective of a *practicing* primary care physician. There comes a point in our lives when we just have to say what is on our minds. And in 2012 I hit that point. I have written fiction before, some of it published, and I wrote a fairly extensive thesis on health care delivery in college, but since then my career has been anything but academic. You may say that I am a down and dirty doctor living in the trenches; I work seeing patients five days a week, often ten hours a day, while I am on call 24/7 365 days a year, typically answering messages continuously throughout the day, including immediately before turning off my lights at night and immediately after tuning them on in the morning, and sometimes in between. I am the medical director of a few long-term care facilities, I run a busy practice, and my computer is on day and night and through the weekend, whether I am preparing talks that I give weekly to nurses and patients, or deciphering Medicare's new rules, or completing notes or other mandatory tasks, or putting my practice's financial house in order. In my opinion all of these roles and responsibilities make me singularly qualified to offer insight into geriatric health care delivery and the role of Medicare. But whenever I pick up a newspaper, watch TV, listen to the radio, or attend a conference, no one like me ever utters a word. Rather we hear from self-proclaimed "experts"—doctors with the title of professor, academics who see patients rarely and whose focus is elsewhere, health care economists, media personalities, politicians—some of whom may have earned the right to put MD after their name, but none of whom has the hard-knocks experience and pragmatic knowledge that so many of us practicing primary care doctors possess. So, that is why I decided to write a book. Working primary care doctors have been left in the dark for too long, and because of that the entire system has suffered.

My professional journey began in Massachusetts, when my wife and I left Charlottesville, Virginia, after completing our Internal Medicine residencies, with our six-month-old son in tow. I joined a small practice in Taunton, an experience that taught me how to be a doctor. Two years later, a second son now added to our family, we moved to Columbia, Maryland, to the house in which we still live, and truly began our professional careers. I joined a five-doctor practice at a retirement community, a wonderful job in which I would spend the next fifteen years. We had a beautiful daughter and watched our three children thrive, and along the way I grew as a geriatric physician. Five years ago I decided to start my own practice, primarily because I wanted to be my own boss and practice medicine my own way. To a large extent, that is exactly how it has played out, with bumps along the way, many of them placed by the very "experts" who contend they are "fixing" our health care system. And as my practice has grown, and my responsibilities have expanded, I am fully immersed in the geriatric health care delivery system. That is when I started to sense a disturbing disconnect between what all the experts in health care were saying from their academic and intellectual perches, and what I and my primary care colleagues were experiencing in the real world that exists far beneath their perceptions.

The Affordable Care Act (ACA or Obamacare) and novel reforms being heralded by Medicare promised a great deal to those of us in primary care. From my perspective, these programs heralded a new appreciation of primary care; all the experts touted primary care doctors as the most important linchpins of any successful health care reform. Even our president discussed primary care in only the most glowing light. But then reality set in. More paperwork, more regulations, new mandatory programs that were time-consuming and expensive, the threat of government audits with potentially large fines; all of this struck us hard in primary care, and all had been engineered by "experts" in the name of reform. Doctors dropped out of Medicare, others (concierge doctors) eliminated insurance completely and charged patients a fee. Hospitals started buying small practices that could not otherwise survive. Workloads increased and overhead costs escalated, most of it not related to patient care. Many of us feared for our futures. One doctor who sits high in ladder of CMS (the Centers for Medicare and Medicaid Services) told me that practices like mine would essentially be extinct in the next five years. And so I wondered why there was such a large gap between what the experts were promising us and what the reformers were actually delivering to us. In reality I knew the answer. And that is what started filling the pages of my book.

A wave of discontent has been simmering in primary care, and much of that has found its way into my book. Two Daily Beast articles from April, 2014 highlight what many of us in the trenches have known for a long time.[12] Begins one of the articles: "Doctors are miserable, patients are miserable, and there's no end in sight. It's time to revamp the healthcare system from the ground up—starting with primary care." The article contends that health care delivery has been co-opted by "thought leaders" including academics, consultants, and policy experts, while 82 percent of practicing physicians like me "feel powerless to influence the profession." One primary care doctor interviewed, who supports a movement to drop out of insurance completely and simply charge patients a membership fee, states that the system is so broken that it cannot be fixed. "'I always say you can't polish a turd. That's what most pundits and consultants are trying to do: hence the advent of Accountable Care Organizations (ACO's) and patient centered medical home constructs. These do nothing to address the culture. They simply impose more restrictions, mandates, and parameters on dangerously stretched physicians." This is a sentiment with which many of us who practice medicine absolutely agree.

The author states that nine out of ten doctors discourage others from joining the profession, and that many "doctors feel that America has declared war on physicians—and both physicians and patients are losers." The ACA has codified a system where primary care doctors are the workhorses with no power to impact change. They are judged by productivity and patient satisfaction scores, which have little relevance to quality care. "But the primary care doctor doesn't have the political power to say no to anything—so the 'to do' list continues to lengthen. A stunning and unmanageable number of forms...show up on a physician's desk needing to be signed. Reams of lab results, refill requests, emails, and callbacks pop up continually on the computer screen. Calls to plead to insurance companies are peppered throughout the day. Every decision carries with it an implied threat of malpractice litigation. Failing to attend to these things brings prompt disciplining or patient complaint. And mercilessly, all of these tasks have to be done on the exhausted doctor's personal time." To me this is an ideal description of a good day; what I love about practicing medicine—spending time with my patients—often takes a back seat to the meaningless busywork we are told me must complete, much of it driven by the ACA and Medicare's reforms. Concludes the article: "To be sure many people with good intentions are working toward solving the healthcare crisis. But the answers they've come up with are driving up costs and driving out doctors."

When I completed my book in the winter of 2013, and I wrote a query letter to send to editors, I decided to try my luck with the academic press. I was elated that almost immediately I heard from the editor of a major university-affiliated press, which happened to be the home of some of the most forward thinking academic doctors involved in health care delivery research. After reading my manuscript and talking to me a few times, she gave me the good news in March of 2013 "I am very pleased to let you know that we would like to offer you an advanced contract for your book." She told me that an academic reviewer would look over the book and recommend changes, and that she would send me the contract within a few weeks.

A month later, while I was at the Chesapeake Bay for spring break with my wife and daughter, the editor emailed me again. The academic reviewer, it turns out, slammed the book, and because of that the editor withdrew her contract. The reviewer stated that while at a recent conference of medical directors he learned, in contrast to my book's allegations, that in fact CMS was reforming geriatric health care, and that I was out of touch. "A speaker from CMS spoke about a multitude of programs funded through the Innovation center. Real change is happening. There are robust models of Accountable Care Organizations and Medicare is simply not headed for Dr. Lazris' simplistic model of co-pays for specialists," he wrote, expressing a sentiment that contradicts my own experience with Medicare reform and that of other working primary care doctors whose real-world experiences are relayed in forums such as the *Daily Beast* articles that I cited above. It was clear from some of his comments that he had not even read my book beyond perhaps a few lines here and there. Ironically, another practicing geriatric physician friend and I were at the same conference and left with just the opposite impression than did this academic reviewer, who seemed to have no real understanding of these innovations and how they impacted us in primary care. I fully knew that it was not I who was out of touch. But it was he who was judging me and latching on to Medicare's new reforms as some theoretical savior.

The editor, who still wanted to publish my book, worked with me in "fixing" it. We changed the structure, added references, and sharpened the themes. I spent the entire summer working on the manuscript; my son helped me with literature searches, and I dug up hundreds of articles I had read. By October I was able to send the new draft back to the editor. She responded: "The revised manuscript is excellent—you did a great job—it's much tighter, more focused, and very powerful throughout." She promised to find better reviewers this time. It took her a while, and I received my verdict in January 2014

The first two reviewers had some reservations, primarily with regard to the book's audience and marketability, but overall had favorable comments. One of them wrote: "I thoroughly enjoyed reading this manuscript. The scholarship is thorough and largely accurate. He writes clearly, is well organized and uses case examples appropriately to illustrate his thesis." The second one wrote: "Superior documentation with a mix of the very newest coming out of the geriatric literature as well as more classical references over the past two decades…He is on target, and this material, which is reaching a small readership of geriatric physicians, needs to gain prominence in both clinical practice and national discussions."

The third reviewer, however, was not as kind. From the first word of his critique, he hammered the book, calling it crass, abrasive, unprofessional, and offensive, the very antithesis of a good academic book. "Dr. Lazris' manuscript reads primarily as a denunciation of the care of the elderly in America, as he perceives it, as well as prolific criticisms and attacks on the current medical establishment, Medicare, physicians, hospitals, the pharmaceutical industry, politicians, hospice, and the general public." Much of his review was even harsher than that. At that point, the editor dropped me from consideration.

However hurt and offended I was by the review, and by my entire unsatisfactory experience with this academic publisher, it did wake me up to a certain reality. Many academic doctors, such as the ones who had decimated my book, live in a very different world than I and so many of my hardworking primary care colleagues. These are the people who make policy, who study health care delivery from their stuffy offices, who advocate the new reforms without having actually experienced them, and then who ultimately judge us. When studies show that 82 percent of practicing physicians feel powerless to influence our profession, it is because people like this bury us under their theoretical constructs and fail to involve us in any reform. In fact, they would probably be very averse to tasting our reality, because that would disrupt the neat and simplistic perceptions to which many of them blindly adhere.

I sent my query letter to a couple of mainstream publishers, but without a professorial title or any expert status, I fully knew that it would end up in someone's trash. That is when one of my patients told me to self-publish; he had done it before, and he felt that Amazon was better than an established publishing house. Others with whom I spoke agreed. At that point, my decision was made.

In truth, this is not an academic book, as much as it is supported by evidence and research. It is a book reflective of a brewing anger among those of us who actually practice geriatric primary care, those of us who have been trampled on and muffled. It is a story seen through my experienced eyes, however jaded they may be. Perhaps it is a bit crass, perhaps it may offend. But in many of our opinions, the academic, political, and policy communities have let us down, and we in primary care have been stranded. As copious "reforms" are thrust on our laps, hampering us from effectively taking care of our patients, we know that there is a better way. My book is an attempt by a practicing primary care doctor to lend a voice to the Medicare debate. It is incredulous to us that we are not driving the entire process and instead are left in the shadow of others. But my hope is that a certain truth will emerge from these pages, and the public will no longer be willing to accept the status quo. Those who script policy often do not know what is really transpiring within the world that they are trying to change, and this book s largely devoted to revealing that hidden truth. Until they know what is wrong in the current world of geriatric health care delivery, something that we in primary care live with every day, it is not possible for anyone to make it right. The machine that drives us can either facilitate what we do or stand in our way, and right now it teeters on the brink of doing neither. It is up to us in primary care, and the patients for whom we care, to make our voices known and influence the conversation.

Andy Lazris, MD
May 28, 2014
Columbia, MD

# INTRODUCTION

## MY BOSS

"Nearly all men die of their remedies and not of their illnesses."
Moliere, *Le Malade Imaginaire*, 1673

Recently I gave an educational talk to a group of nurses and aides at a nursing home and assisted-living facility about the dangers of hospitalizing the frail elderly who live in long-term care. I am a certified medical director (CMD), which means that I took courses and other extensive training to acquire a title that I can tack on after my MD. But most significantly, through my training and subsequent conferences I learned how to be a medical director of long-term care facilities, mastering the regulatory minutiae and Medicare rules that impact much of geriatric medicine in the twenty-first century. I currently direct several assisted-living facilities, retirement communities, and a nursing home. When I talk to the nursing staff, I usually focus on a pragmatic arena of health care that will alter the way they care for their aged patients.

In this talk I distributed a handout elucidating the many pitfalls that elderly people may encounter in a hospital, highlighting the lack of efficacy and inherent dangers of hospital care in many circumstances. In fact, as I hammered multiple times in my talk, treating them in the facility itself is typically more humane and beneficial. The talk went over particularly well, as the nurses and aides understood the futility of hospitalization from their ample experience and enjoyed discussing the topic.

However later that night I received notice that one of the nurses who attended the talk sent a ninety-eight-year-old demented woman from the assisted-living facility to the hospital for confusion and weakness. At the hospital the woman became more confused and had to be sedated. She had needles shoved into her arm and was tossed in a head scan, something that must have been frightening to her. She also was exposed to harmful medicines, to dangerous infections, to a high likelihood of treatment mistakes, and to a medical system that pushes the most aggressive of care on elderly people despite a paucity of evidence to support that approach. As is common, they found a urine infection (something fairly ubiquitous in the elderly, to which much illness is ascribed) and they sent her back, not admitting her to the hospital where she may have been tied down and exposed to even more deleterious trauma.

I was somewhat irritated that within hours of hearing my talk on hospitalization, a nurse still insisted on sending this confused patient to the hospital for a fairly common medical issue, when I believed that the patient would have been better off staying put and having more gentle care and observation in familiar surroundings. But I understood all the many forces that conspired to force her to do something that likely she did not think was clinically necessary or even prudent, something we will discuss extensively in this book.

I saw the patient a few days later. She was in a room with other demented residents, sitting in a chair, smiling, and clapping her hands. Some of the nursing aides were leading them in a sing-along. At that moment, freed from blood pressure cuffs, blood sticks, x-ray machines, nursing home regulatory rules, and handfuls of medicine, my patient was receiving perfect geriatric care. She was socializing, exercising, and using her brain. She was under no stress. She was not exposed to the sting of modern medicine. The dichotomy between her experience at the hospital and what I witnessed now was striking to me. Now she was in the hands of people who knew her and were making her life enjoyable, instead of at the mercy of people who dug into her elderly body trying to find problems and fix them. The former scenario is the very epitome of good geriatric care, the latter is a geriatrician's nightmare. The former is also cheap and humane, while the latter is horribly expensive, tearing our Medicare system to shreds while decimating its unknowing victims. Unfortunately, it is the latter that is becoming the norm in the geriatric wilderness that I inhabit. And the most tragic part is that Medicare itself is financing and encouraging the very aggressive care that is its own dagger.

With this book I hope to demonstrate how our health care system is failing our oldest and frailest Americans, and how that failure is inextricably tied to Medicare's philosophy and payment structure. An idea has blossomed within our medical thinking that equates aggressive, specialized care with good care, even for patients very advanced in years. That lore has taken root in how Medicare treats its seniors, and prompts our financially strapped national insurance to thrust a large amount of its budget into futile efforts to keep people alive at the end of their lives with the full gamut of technologically advanced medical services. But very little evidence exists to support the utility of what many people label as "thorough" care in the elderly. For those of us who practice medicine every day, we in fact know otherwise.

I am an internist, and the focus of my practice has been on geriatrics, caring for the old. I love the idea of Medicare. I studied it as a history student at Brown University, and I have been immersed in it for the past twenty-five years. During my professional life I have read the debates in Congress and among the intellectual elites about its future, have listened to the politicians and academic giants dissect its flaws, have studied Medicare's own solutions to its woes, and read how the lay press perceives its impending collapse and how it may be saved. But more significantly, every day I live under the shadow of its rules, regulations, and reimbursement. I know Medicare better than anyone, because it is my perpetual companion; it is my boss. So as I listen to the people in ivory towers talk about Medicare on the pages of the *Washington Post* or the sound waves of NPR, as I hear CMS representatives and geriatric academic leaders talk with wonder about the new innovations that are around the corner, I just cringe, wondering what they are seeing that seems so different to me. True, I am just a doctor, and not one with any more titles and credentials than caring for patients affords me. But I do understand Medicare. I know why it is failing, and how it can be saved. And it comes down to acknowledging what really is Medicare's philosophy and how that thinking has led Medicare down a precarious path.

Because I am a geriatric physician, Medicare controls a huge part of my life. It pays the bills and sets the rules of my practice. I cannot charge more or less than it dictates to me, I must write notes as it instructs, and even my interactions with families and patients are controlled by its regulations. Medicare is truly my boss. And Medicare is not without its bosses. The consumers of health care—my patients—hold Medicare's reins, because Medicare ultimately rewards those who utilize its resources the most, and neglects those who age with dignity and comfort. Many can, and do, exhaust the system's finances with an interminable search for eternal life. Some believe a false credo that more is better, fueled in their misconception by doctors, the press, drug companies, and the very zeitgeist of the American way of life. Others are pushed to be aggressive by Medicare's rules. Hovering over everything is the politics of perception: when Medicare curtails any service, people on both sides of the political aisle cry foul, insinuating that any restriction in Medicare's quest to do everything for everyone is akin to letting our elderly die. It is difficult to reform Medicare under such a toxic cloud.

There is a national obsession with illness in our county. Americans think they are sick and perpetually search for cure and resolution,[3] especially as they age. Their quest for medical answers to the ravages of aging fills them with a heavy dose of stress, merely exacerbating their own decline and dragging the health care delivery system down with them.[4] [5] The public—from patients and their families to doctors and experts and politicians and journalists—perceive that more is better in regards to caring for the elderly. And they believe that with enough perseverance, our health care delivery system is capable of virtually anything, even reversing the ravages of aging. Those are Medicare's bosses, and

Medicare rewards them by financing their plunge into a sea of aggressive care. It is because of all these bosses that Medicare is about to lose its wheels.

This book is essentially about the very old. One could argue that the youngest and most vibrant Medicare recipients, many of whom still work and engage in vigorous activity, may benefit from aggressive care. There are many who dispute this claim, but I will not try to address that debate in my book. Most of my subjects are the oldest and sickest of our Medicare patients, many who have dementia, many who live in assisted-living facilities and nursing homes, and who often utilize excessive Medicare resources without deriving any benefit from their "thorough" care. To what would actually help the very old—compassionate care delivered in their own homes—Medicare turns its blind eye, reluctant to assist those who seek dignity and comfort in their quest to stay healthy and active in their later years without being shoved into the claws of medical excess.

A century or so ago American medicine evolved from a field dominated by charlatans who dispensed potions and false promises to a distinguished profession led by well-trained practitioners versed in the science of medical care. (See Paul Starr's *The Social Transformation of American Medicine* for an excellent discussion of the history of health care in America.) Unfortunately, as medical science advanced, so too did the perception that science and technology could cure everything. More machines, drugs, procedures, and tests sprouted across our medical landscape, and a lore grew that all illness, even the illness of age itself, would fall prey to the ingenuity of American medicine. People no longer had to get sick and die. By utilizing all of our brilliant resources, by assaulting disease at its roots, we could halt the aging process and begin a trek toward immortality. None of that proved to be true, but the public started to believe it. More specialists emerged, promising more narrowly focused care. More scans, more drugs, and bigger and more sophisticated hospitals all sprouted across the landscape, growing from an errant belief. And into this landscape stepped Medicare, the most expansive leap into health care delivery ever enacted by the US government.

President Truman first attempted to create a comprehensive, inclusive health care system that ultimately was drowned by a perception, despised in America, that his reform would lead to rationing of care,[6] a fate that destroyed President Clinton's attempted reform efforts and emasculated President Obama's ACA, all for similar reasons. When President Johnson pushed through Medicare in 1965, he too met vigorous opposition from medical and community groups that feared a loss of autonomy for patients and doctors and envisioned that Medicare would spark a socialized medical system that would decimate America's medical excellence and lead to rationing. The AMA (American Medical Association) especially fought to stop Medicare's enactment,[7][8][9][10][11] something I researched as part of my senior thesis at Brown University. I pored through AMA journals, in which physicians and medical experts predicted doom if Medicare became reality, and I read contemporary articles in newspapers and magazines that mirrored much of the debate that we are hearing now regarding health care reform and its potential to destroy quality through rationing. The AMA actually proposed its own more private insurance plan for the elderly called Eldercare even as it threatened to boycott Medicare and not participate. When it finally did agree to endorse Medicare, the AMA had forced enough concessions from the government, especially with regard to keeping hospitals strong and independent, that it actually gained financially from the plan's enactment.[12][13][14][15] It is not ironic, then, that the AMA is one of many medical organizations now fighting to keep Medicare intact and largely unchanged, despite its initial opposition to the plan. Doctors and hospitals thrive in Medicare, as Medicare finances the most advanced and aggressive medical care for all elderly Americans. At Medicare's birth such a philosophy seemed both sound and affordable. But the medical profession, and the population it serves, has changed dramatically since 1965.

When Medicare was envisioned, there were far fewer elderly in America requiring health care. The population over age 65, before

Medicare started caring for them, accounted for about 8 percent of the population, or twelve million people. By 2009 the elderly represented 12.8 percent of the population, tripling to thirty-five million people. By 2050 the elderly are expected to be 20 percent of the US population, exploding to 88.5 million people. Of the elderly, the very old are proportionately growing faster than any other group. Those over eighty are projected to be the most populous age group by 2050, representing 7.4 percent of the population, or 32.5 million people.[16] Medicare must now serve more and older people than its framers anticipated.

The number of Medicare recipients with diseases of dementia, such as Alzheimer's disease, has also ballooned since the insurance's inception. At the time Medicare was scripted, Alzheimer's was not even identified as a medical condition, and the cost of dementia care was minimal. But as that reality has changed, the cost of such care has accelerated rapidly. Currently five million Americans are diagnosed as having Alzheimer's, and that number is expected to reach seven million by 2025. The cost of caring for those people is estimated at $203 billion, over half of which is paid by Medicare. That number is expected to reach $1.2 trillion by 2050.[17] Health care costs for US residents with dementia are triple the cost of other nondemented elderly, approximately $33,000 per recipient per year versus $10,000 for those without dementia.[18] Currently sixty-one million Americans care for their ill or disabled family members, many of whom have dementia, spending an average of eighteen hours a week doing so. A quarter of the baby boom generation provides care for an aging parent.[19] Because Medicare pays so little to help care for demented people in their homes, often families have to resort to hospitalizing their loved ones out of desperation, something that escalates Medicare costs needlessly. Medicare's framers never considered the consequences of dementia and other debilitating diseases of aging on its model of care.

In addition to the sheer numbers and illnesses of its clients, Medicare's expenses are impacted by changes in health care delivery since 1965. We are now a medical society dominated by specialists, high-priced tests and procedures, and very expensive hospitals. Compared to 1965, Medicare patients now have at their disposal massive amounts of medical technology that society has embraced as being the most thorough means of assaulting illness and disability. In addition, because the AMA persuaded Medicare to focus on and finance hospital care above all else, every American over age sixty-five has access to Medicare A, which pays for hospitalization. The hospital is free for all elderly Americans after a single deductible (approximately $1,000), a cost that is usually paid by their secondary insurance. The hospital remains the center of care for the elderly, the place where older Americans must flock when they are too sick to stay at home, when they seek Medicare's payment for round-the-clock nursing and rehabilitation services, and when they want Medicare to pay for certain invasive treatments such as IV fluids and antibiotics. Under Medicare's current payment structure, the frail elderly are pushed into the hospital even when they would prefer to stay at home, despite the peril and price tag that such a journey entails.

Medicare B covers most other services, including doctor's visits, tests, procedures, and physical therapy. Americans have to pay a small premium to enroll in Medicare B, and well over 90 percent of Americans have done this. After charging patients a nominal deductible (approximately $150), Medicare B will pay for 80 percent of all services. The vast majority of Americans purchase secondary insurance that will pay the 20 percent of cost that Medicare does not cover. Thus, most elderly Americans, after paying their annual premiums and deductible, will get all medical services without charge. Medicare B will not pay for meaningful health care in the home, for home health aides, or for medicines. Often when they get too ill patients will need to use Medicare A, and that typically requires a stay in the hospital. In its current rendition, Medicare puts no limits on expensive tests and specialty visits, encourages hospitalization for those most ill, and does not contribute to more palliative care in the home.

The newest incarnation of Medicare that was enacted in 2006, Medicare D, covers a large part of medication costs for those recipients who pay an annual fee. Already by 2010 the program was costing the federal government $62 billion, or 12 percent of the entire Medicare budget.[20] Congress made two crucial errors in enacting part D. First, it underestimated the cost of the program and how widely it would be used. Second, it explicitly forbade the government from negotiating with pharmaceutical companies to create a formulary of reasonably priced medicines, a strategy that other federal agencies such as the VA have employed to keep costs down. As a result, Medicare D recipients can choose the most expensive brand-name drugs with little restriction and with no competitive price reductions.[21] In our medical landscape cluttered by high-priced drugs that promise miraculous results to the elderly, Medicare D has become an albatross that strangles the entire Medicare system.

The result of Medicare's failure to adjust as the world has changed around it has taken a toll on the US economy, placing Medicare under the political microscope as one of the primary drivers of our budget deficit. While Medicare represented 2 percent of federal spending in 1970, it jumped to 15 percent by 2011,[22] due to the aging of our population and the increasing cost of medical care. Although over the past few years the rate of growth of Medicare has slowed, it is still growing and becoming more costly. The financial numbers are staggering. Medicare cost the government $7.1 billion in 1970, $35 billion in 1980, $109.7 billion in 1990, $219 billion in 2000, and $550 billion in 2012.[23] The cost of care escalates for the oldest of Medicare's recipients. In 2008 the per capita cost among Medicare recipients over eighty-five was nearly double the amount spent by younger people. ($13,219 versus $7,626). The cost of those who reported that they were in poor health was even higher, $22,612. Many of these people are very old, demented, and live in institutions.[24] Many of them are forced into the hospital and encouraged to undergo tests and procedures that are both costly and ineffective. No amount of money can fix their aging bodies, and much of the money thrust at them likely only causes more harm, as we will show. A recent *Washington Post* article highlighted that in the American medical system

1 percent of patients exhaust 21 percent of total health care costs, at a price of $88,000/person/year.[25] Clearly the sickest Americans, many of whom are not likely to improve despite the money spent on their care are taxing our system, often for reasons instigated by Medicare itself.

Can thorough and aggressive medical care help prolong life and improve quality in our oldest patients? The very idea that an overutilization of health care leads to improved outcomes has been debunked repeatedly,[26] [27] something we will explore extensively in this book. We in the geriatric field know it innately; our very souls are watered by the knowledge that more is less, and that aggressive care can be deleterious care. When one studies the literature it becomes apparent that there is a paucity of data specifically relevant to our oldest patients, many of whom have multiple illnesses and are on a plethora of medicines.[28] [29] So, often erroneously, we extrapolate data from younger patients, or we make assumptions that have been hammered into our heads, that all diseases should be eradicated, and that our society is blessed with an abundance of life-saving treatments. In fact, as little as 15 percent of what doctors do is backed up by valid evidence.[30] And thus do we send our oldest and frailest patients on a journey that is costly to both them and to society with little evidence to back us up.

Many books and studies have explored the false notion that aggressive care leads to improved outcome in the elderly, and I have been lucky enough to be able to use them as resources. These include:

- Nortin Hadler, *The Last Well Person* and *Rethinking Aging*
- H. Gilbert Welch, *Overdiagnosed*
- Shannon Brownlee, *Overtreated*
- John Abramson, *Over-dosed America*
- Erik Rifkin, *The Illusion of Certainty*
- Robert Duggan, *Breaking the Iron Triangle*
- Ira Byock, *The Best Care Possible* and other books
- Multiple studies by Jack Wennberg and Elliott Fisher regarding their work with the Wennberg Institute at Dartmouth College

But the crux of my argument flows from my own experience and that of my colleagues. While medical literature can help guide us to make sensible decisions, most of us who practice medicine every day have become skeptical as to the validity of what we read in journals. We know that many studies are financed by pharmaceutical companies and special interest groups, that the overly screened subjects accepted into such studies look nothing like the more complicated patients we see every day, and that the conclusions are subject to many interpretations. We also have seen studies touting the benefits of a drug or treatment, only to be completely reversed some years later. When I was a medical student it was considered standard of care to treat women with estrogen after menopause, and it was deemed to be dangerous to treat patients with failing hearts (congestive heart failure) with a class of drugs called beta blockers. Studies and literature supported such suppositions, academic physicians assured us of their validity, and clinical pathways enshrined such beliefs as gospel. Well, some years later, new studies emerged, and now it is bad practice to give women estrogen after menopause, or to deny patients with congestive heart failure beta blocker drugs. There are so many examples where science and dogma are thrown on their heads, leaving us doctors to ascertain reality for ourselves. Also, I have seen academics and physicians interpret a single study to argue opposite points, showing me that the literature is far less scientific and objective than we are led to believe. Finally, few large studies focus on the frail elderly among their subjects, and those are the people most vulnerable to the sting of aggressive care. Hence, my book, while citing the literature that is out there, relies on my own experience as a geriatric doctor to reach many of its conclusions.

What drives Medicare's continued advocacy of aggressive medical care despite its suffocating cost and lack of efficacy? And why are draconian measures not being taken to curb that excess and to redefine geriatric medical care so that it can sensibly address the changing population that it serves?

At present we live in a specialized medical society where technology is king. Hospitals, certain doctors, and many institutions benefit from aggressive care. Drug companies too. By denying "thorough" care to the most frail of our elderly, many doctors and institutions would be financially hurt. Thus, a strong wall of opposition stands against the thrust of meaningful change.

My most frail patients, and their families, also often demand "thorough" care for many reasons. One is financial; as we will discuss, under Medicare's rules it is often much less expensive for them to get aggressive medical treatment than to be conservative and compassionate, even if it costs Medicare substantially more and the outcomes of such care may be worse. But just as important, many of my oldest patients, and their families who ultimately make their decisions, believe in aggressive care. They have been inundated by the idea that more is better at any age, that numbers need to be fixed, that a cure is out there if only they pursue it. Even those who are skeptical are forced to live in a society where everyone else is telling them to be aggressive. When conservatives talk about death panels, and liberals declare that any restrictions on Medicare spending is akin to killing people, it is difficult for anyone to make rational decisions.

My own life as a doctor has demonstrated to me the futility of pursing excessively thorough care for many elderly patients, while revealing to me the wall that Medicare has enacted preventing us from offering our patients a more sensible and economical alternative. My career started in a small town called Taunton, and that two-year experience opened my eyes wide to what is wrong with our current Medicare system. Taunton was a world unto itself. Small and isolated in the bog-filled serenity of southeastern Massachusetts, speckled with ethnic Portuguese who had been there for generations, Taunton housed a population of working-class families who rarely moved away or thought much beyond the confines of their town. When one of my patients occasionally relocated twenty miles away to the Portuguese enclaves of New Bedford or Fall River, their families mourned their abandonment. And although they lived a half hour away from the medical meccas of Boston and Providence, most of my patients refused to travel that far; they preferred little Morton Hospital with six beds in a room and their spattering of local doctors. They trusted us, they listened to us, they respected us, and they treated us with unfettered kindness.

In Taunton my patients understood the limits of medical intervention. They did not chase medical miracles or rely on the promises made by aggressive doctors, pharmaceuticals, and the press. Compared to the well-educated enclaves in which I practiced subsequently, my Taunton patients understood the aging process and based their decisions on common sense and dignity. These were the smartest group of patients with whom I have ever worked.

Often on my way home to East Providence I made home visits, where I was greeted with a hug and a smile, never a list of demands or piles of Internet articles. One day I stopped to see an elderly Portuguese woman with moderate dementia. She lived in a two-story colonial house that was older than she, cuddled upstairs in a small bedroom with a hospital bed and a large metal lifting mechanism (called a hoyer lift) juxtaposed with some old upholstered furniture and a nightstand. Grandkids ran in and out, up and down; any number of them visited the house regularly. Some children lived in the house, many others lived nearby, all congregated here on the days I arrived.

Whenever I saw Mrs. A. she smiled and held my hands gently. She spit out a few words in Portuguese that her daughters translated for me, typically more niceties than anything of substance. I usually listened as she or her daughters expressed any concerns. We reviewed her medicines, stopping any we could. I took her blood pressure, and waved my stethoscope on her heart and lungs, a requisite action by any of us in the medical field. After my brief visit Mrs. A. thanked me profoundly, typically with a kiss on the cheek, after which her daughter pushed something on me, whether some homemade sweet bread or a box of candy. I always left elated, although part of my brain questioned the significance of the service I provided or why Medicare would pay me for doing so little.

One dreary and cold day in the New England winter I stopped by her house at the behest of one of her daughters. After our traditional greetings, I noticed that Mrs. A.'s eyes were yellow. She was scratching herself, something that proved to be her daughter's only concern. She still smiled, and the stomping and laughter of children had not faded one bit. I examined her. She had a large liver protruding down to her groin, and she was severely jaundiced. I was concerned.

I took her daughter aside. "Your mom has something serious going on," I told her. "She has jaundice. We may need to do some tests."

The daughter smiled. "My mother is eighty-five years old," she said. "If we could just give her something for her itching. She seems so uncomfortable."

"But it could be treatable," I went on. "Maybe it's a gallstone. Or a resectable cancer."

The daughter put her hands on my shoulder. "She is eighty-five," she repeated, with a smile that shined with absolute serenity and conviction. "I don't want to put her through all those tests. But I would like her not to be so uncomfortable, if that is even possible. You tell us what is best."

I nodded and gave her both an antihistamine for the itching and some Questran powder that worked particularly well for the jaundice itch (although very constipating, as I warned the daughter). The daughter stepped to another room for a moment, and returned with a bottle of wine in a weaved basket casing. "Take this," she said. "And thank you. My mother feels so much better after your visits. And so does the whole family. Thank you so much." It was if the daughter knew that this would be my final visit.

Mrs. A. died many months later, comfortable and surrounded by her family.

If only all of our country followed the sensible script of Mrs. A. and Taunton. She charged Medicare no more than the cost of a few of my visits and some rented medical supplies. Probably less than a thousand dollars. And all of this for the perfect ending to a stress-free aging process.

Contrast that to a child who chided me for not checking her eighty-plus-year-old dad's PSA blood test, and when she did bring him to a urologist at a major academic medical center to perform that test, and it showed that he had prostate cancer, she graced me with several instructional notes about how his new squadron of doctors were actually doing something for her dad, rather than neglecting him as I did. After a multitude of tests, biopsies, scans, treatments, and visits to the most brilliant minds at the mecca of medical science, as my once carefree patient became consumed by a cauldron of stress, he finally did die, of a heart attack, not anything to do with his PSA. To which his child said: "At least I know that they were thorough in their treatment of my dad and we did all we could to get him well." She would have had it no other way. Tens of thousands of dollars later, dollars paid by Medicare, her father died of stress, likely precipitated by the very misguided pursuit that Medicare financed.

In any given week I may encounter a patient or family member who demands unreasonable tests, treatments, hospitalizations, specialist visits, and impossible answers for the ravages of aging in patients little different than Mrs. A. And instead of loving kindness and an acceptance of aging, they conjure incessant stress for themselves, their loved ones, and me and my staff by trying to achieve the impossible. On any given day I will encounter many more patients and families who prefer to live the life of Mrs. A., to be kept comfortable, to be on fewer medicines and have fewer tests, but who are pushed reluctantly in the direction of aggressive care by a medical system, a society, and an insurance that enables and encourages excess.

Whenever I hear about proposals to ameliorate our society's excessive consumption of medical care, I find that many reformers ascribe blame to doctors who both profit from and relish a health care system that is fueled by excess. They concoct ingenious theories that contend that by tying physician salary to performance and not to fee-for-service, somehow patients will no longer be allowed to abuse services. But in my career I have seen it from a different angle. Many primary care doctors do their best to stop older patients from pursing aggressive care, only to be met by a system that not only pays for that care but encourages it. In fact, we as primary care physicians have no capacity to slow the overuse of resources. Medicare encourages patients and families to be aggressive, and it pays specialists and hospitals generously to be aggressive; we often just get in the way.

One of my good friends, a fellow geriatric physician, lamented to me the other day about a situation involving a patient of his, Mrs. L., far more ill than Mrs. A. She was old and demented, although independent just a few months ago until she was pummeled by a series of medical insults that left her weak and nursing home bound. She needed kidney dialysis and artificial food to keep her alive. My friend was appalled to learn that her family sought to pursue every option and treatment to maintain her life at all costs, even though several doctors had advised them otherwise. "She was living on her own just a few months ago," her family members said. My friend spent hours of unreimbursed time talking to doctors, reviewing notes, and reasoning with her children. But they persevered. "She was living on her own just a few months ago." They could not get past that fact. And the more my friend pushed to keep her comfortable, the more they resisted him. So they found a new doctor, one willing to perform dialysis on a woman who could no longer feed herself or talk, dialysis that is well reimbursed by Medicare. And they found a new nursing home willing to endorse their aggressive approach to care.

These were educated children. One was a nurse. But how little they understood the aging process, and how little they realized what older people really desire in their last months. Over 70 percent of elderly say they want to die at home, not in a hospital.[31] But there is a very sharp divide between the more palliative approach that most elderly seek and how aggressively their families, doctors, and the system treats them.[32] [33] [34] [35] Many families are peering through a jaded lens. They love their mom so much that they just want to keep her alive and wish for a miracle, the miracle of reversing age and returning her to her healthy state when she lived alone. The illusion of turning back the clock with aggressive care is alluring but often deceptive. In the elderly, it only takes one illness to trigger a chain reaction in the body that decimates it. Healthy three months ago and dialysis dependent now does not mean a mere blip has occurred. It is rather one of the consequences of aging, the end stage of a process that was accelerating beneath the surface and then exploded to its tragic conclusion. But fantasy overtakes their thoughts. Medicare pays the bills. And their mom pays the price.

Many of my patients squander tens of thousands of Medicare dollars in their last months of life, clinging to a quixotic hope that cure is possible if you push hard enough and spend enough money. End-of-life expenses, in fact, are one of the primary drivers of medical costs for the elderly. Twenty-five percent of total Medicare expenses finance end-of-life care, care that accomplishes nothing but painfully prolonging the inevitable. Incredibly, with the full endorsement of Medicare, the health care profession tosses the gamut of its medical resources at problems that are not able to be fixed and merely lead to death.[36][37][38][39][40] While only a negligible amount of Medicare funds are spent on helping people like Mrs. A. stay comfortable in their home where they can receive appropriate medical care, Medicare spends a quarter of its entire budget trying to save people who are not savable.

Although a majority of elderly people want to die at home with comfort, only a fifth of them actually achieve that goal. Fifty percent die in a hospital, and 40 percent of those are in intensive care units "where they will likely be sedated or have their arms tied down." Few elderly elect to be treated with such flagrantly ineffective aggression in their final days and months, but many forces, including the harsh reality of Medicare, push them where they do not want to be. Another 30 percent of the elderly die in nursing homes, often explicitly against their wishes,[41] forced to bow to the financial realities of our current geriatric health care system.

Unless we curb the dangerous folly of aggressive care in our oldest residents, unless we realize that with age comes a decline that no amount of dollars will curtail, unless we stop financing a medical quest that leads to nothing more than the very death it is attempting to stop, then Medicare will not persevere. Few of the innovations concocted by

CMS or the Medicare reformers confront that reality. Few of them are proposing feasible means of helping Mrs. A.'s experience to become the norm.

My book is about all the bosses out there—patients, families, doctors, hospitals, drug companies, facilities, lawyers, newspapers, laws and regulations, and the misplaced dogma so prevalent in our society that more is better. My twenty-five-year experience practicing geriatric medicine has taught me the value of life in its last years, and it has provided me with tocsins of what can go wrong once the illusion of excess obfuscates a clear view of the aging process. When I listen to the debates raging about Medicare among administrators, politicians, and intellectual giants, I realize that they just don't get it. When I am forced to contend with the reforms that the ACA and CMS have tossed at me to curb costs, I realize that they just don't get it. They can pontificate all they want, they can speculate and theorize and argue until they are red in the face, they can throw up graphs and charts and statistics, and blame the doctors for perpetrating waste, but they don't get it. I have always said that if you throw fifty primary care physicians in a room, doctors of every ethnicity and political slant, and ask us to fix Medicare, we would be done well before lunch, although we would likely stay long enough to enjoy a nice lunch if someone else was paying. We would hand you a paper, probably less than a page long, and would tell you it's as simple as that. Because it really is. Once you are out there and live in the shadow of Medicare, it doesn't take a brain surgeon to figure it all out. In fact, the last thing you want is for a brain surgeon to try to figure it all out.

With this book I hope to demonstrate why Medicare is failing and how to effectively fix it, while showing how the beauty of aging can be so dangerously poisoned by allowing the status quo to persevere. Not everyone is Mrs. A. But that is who the system should be rewarding, and right now it is doing just the opposite. And unless it changes course, Medicare will not be as fortunate as Mrs. A.; it will die a difficult and costly death.

# 1

# DEFINING QUALITY: THE QUEST FOR NUMERICAL PERFECTION

*"Everyone dies of something. Every time a new complication develops,*
*the doctor will assign it to a name, giving you another diagnosis...*
*Each diagnosis has a potential treatment, which the doctors will dutifully*
*tell you about—if you haven't already looked it up on line."*
Byock, *The Best Care Possible*

The pharmaceutical industry has thrived in this country because people believe that medicines are both essential and useful to repair a variety of dangerous and bothersome conditions, something that is especially true in the elderly. Whether treating aberrant numbers (blood pressure, cholesterol, sugar, etc.), or helping to resolve nuisance conditions like urinary incontinence and confusion, drugs flood our elderly patients' bodies. But many medications have dubious efficacy and can be frankly dangerous. Very often they are used to treat problems that do not meaningfully improve, and more often they instigate troublesome symptoms, drug interactions, and harmful side effects.

Medicare does not itself compel patients to take more medicines; our national drug obsession is a much more complex phenomenon than can be ascribed simply to Medicare. But especially since the advent of Medicare D and the adaption of clinical performance measures (labed as quality indicators by CMS) to grade doctor quality, Medicare is playing a larger role in encouraging and financing excessive medication use. And as we discussed, Medicare D places minimal restrictions on what drugs patients can take, and does not negotiate with pharmaceutical companies to secure medicines that are lower in cost but equally efficacious. Said one doctor who has studied this problem: "If the government's real goal were to increase senior citizens' access to the most effective medicine, its first step would have been to determine the best care based on the best scientific evidence available, helping patients and doctors to make informed decisions. Instead, the medicine prescription drug bill simply opens the public coffers to pay for price for expensive brand name drugs."[42]

As significantly, Medicare as part of its reform effort is grading doctors based on the quality of their care, something that also can actually lead to more medication use. Through two programs primarily—PQRS and Accountable Care Organizations (ACOs), both of which we will discuss in detail later—Medicare is compelling doctors to produce evidence that they are following quality indicators as defined by CMS. We as physicians are required to complete a preordained set of questions, many of which have very little relevance to our particular patients, and to demonstrate that we are in compliance with a variety of such indicators, something that will eventually help to determine some of what we are paid. It is felt that such pay for performance strategies will help doctors practice better medicine and save the system money. It is a laborious and expensive process for us, and very often it pushes us to mindlessly fill out scripted checklists when our time could be better spent having meaningful discussions with our patients. Since every elderly patient has a unique set of wants and needs, and each one offers unique challenges that make templated responses virtually useless, Medicare's attempt to impose quality standards on us can be more busywork than meaningful change.

Quality indicators have another dark side, one that can increase unnecessary testing and treatment in the elderly. By forcing us to comply with specific standards, Medicare expects us to order tests and prescribe drugs that we, and our patients, may not believe to be beneficial. By tying the quality of our care (and ultimately a portion of our salary) to the achievement of those standards, Medicare is pushing us to act in a way that may actually be counterproductive to quality care. Many indicators are designed to persuade doctors to evaluate and treat abnormal numbers. High blood pressure, high cholesterol, high sugars, abnormal bone density results, low heart ejection fraction, irregular heart rhythms; all of these have specific guidelines that script appropriate testing and treatment. To be fair, many of Medicare's quality indicators are more reasonable than other clinical practice guidelines, many of which seek aggressive care for virtually every abnormal number in the elderly. But virtually none of Medicare's quality guidelines encourage doctors to **avoid** testing for and treating these abnormal numbers even in the very oldest of our patients; at best, they encourage some testing and treating, and are silent about overtreatment. Just how important is it to treat abnormal numbers in the elderly? That is the crux of what we have to explore, for its answer illuminates much of what is wrong with Medicare and how to fix it.

## Numbers

As an internal medicine resident at the University of Virginia, I spent time in a rural clinic in Orange County working with two excellent doctors. One day they sent me to see an old farmer who was in his midnineties and still worked his farm independently. When I saw the man he seemed strong and young, very calm, fairly sharp, and nimble on his feet. I examined him and found nothing particularly wrong except for his blood pressure, which was close to 220/110 from my recollection. To me this finding was startling. I rechecked it a few times, and the results did not change. The man took no medicines and had no serious medical problems. He felt very well.

I talked to one of the clinic doctors and I insisted that we treat the man for his dangerously elevated blood pressure. We had all read the new SHEP study that demonstrated the dangers of high blood pressure in the elderly,[43] and thus we needed to be more vigilant in treating pressure elevations among our older patients. The doctor bucked, but I convinced him to allow me to use a very mild blood pressure medicine, and the patient agreed. I told him that I would go out there next week and check the pressure again. Well, next week never came. Several days after starting the medicine, the man dropped dead. Coincidence? Unlikely. My guess, now that I have more extensive real-life experience with the elderly, is that the man had very narrow arteries to his heart and brain and kidneys, and he needed every bit of that high blood pressure to keep the blood flowing to his vital organs. In fact, his body's natural autoregulation system probably pushed that pressure up to keep him alive. When I gave him a pill to make his numbers look better, I unintentionally dismantled his body's coping mechanism by decreasing that necessary pressure and I instigated his demise.

This is not an isolated event. Number obsession has reached a fever pitch among the elderly and those who care for them. Numbers are everything, even if we are not quite sure what those numbers should be for each individual. As one doctor states in his book on medical excess: America's elderly know their numbers "and are hell bent to be normal."[44] It may be blood pressure, pulse, sugar, cholesterol, kidney function, bone density, thyroid level, blood count, vitamin levels; there is a near infinitude of numbers that can be measured, fussed over, and fixed with medicines. As people age, their numbers deteriorate and verge from what is deemed "normal"; the more we look, the more we will find, and the more medicine we will need to dispense to fix.

We know from science and experience that the aggressive treatment of numerical abnormalities in the elderly, especially in conditions like diabetes and hypertension, frequently causes side effects, worsening physical and mental function, and an impaired quality of life without extending lifespan or even preventing major adverse outcomes (strokes, heart attacks, cancer, etc.) in any measurably significant way. Medicines can fix numbers, but rarely do they improve a geriatric patient's life. In fact, the more we toss into an elderly body, the more interactions and complications will occur. As we will see, low numbers are typically much more immediately dangerous than high ones; I have seen many more people injured and even killed by aggressive treatment that drops their numbers than by benign neglect. But such a reality does not deter the American medical community from employing an army of medication to achieve numerical perfection. If the lore of what defines quality medical care starts anywhere, it is in the theater of medications, where numbers are perceived to be beacons, pills are touted as saviors, and those who push the pills and fix the numbers are our medical saints.

I am frequently told by my patients, or those caring for them, that I have to be more vigilant in monitoring and fixing numbers. Physical therapists and home care nurses e-mail me about blood pressures or sugars that are too high; they often have an alarmist tone when they convey the information, expecting me to intervene quickly. Nursing homes, as we will see, flood us with abnormal numbers that are expected to be fixed, from thyroid levels to blood pressures to sugars to a large variety of labs. They, too—pushed by regulations, unrealistic expectations, and pharmaceutical recommendations—perceive numerical aberrations to be emergencies that require immediate treatments. My patients see specialists, emergency room doctors, and even family members who frighten them about their abnormal numbers. Very often these abnormal numbers are merely blips, taken at inopportune times when patients are in pain, or stressed, or ill. Sometimes the numbers are not even very high, but they have crossed some imaginary line between normal and dangerous. The assumption by many who contact me is that once that line is crossed, then a stroke or heart attack or perhaps even death is imminent.

Since numbers can be incessantly measured, and since so many of them can be "fixed" with medicines, patients often swallow handfuls of pills to push their numbers back to the acceptable side of normal, after which they can be monitored in a variety of ways to assure the numbers stay in line. And if the numbers start to migrate away from what we have deemed to be normal, more medicines and tests will naturally flow through their frail bodies. But what are normal numbers for the elderly, and does fixing abnormal numbers impart any meaningful clinical benefit to our patients?

We can measure numbers many ways. Tests, labs, vital signs: for every patient, we can compile numbers that come to define them. Then we label our patients with diseases that correspond to their errant numbers. They may have high blood pressure, high cholesterol, diabetes, osteoporosis, hypothyroidism, anemia, dementia, and one of any number of conditions that we can treat and then monitor through copious lifelong testing. In my practice the pursuit of numerical excellence is one of the primary reasons that patients see me and an army of specialists on a regular basis. Many doctors who have studied our health care system believe that the medical community is intentionally manufacturing disease by using these numbers because the medical community thrives when more people are sick. Some state that we are turning aging itself into a disease.[45] Having a number that equates to an illness and that can be altered with medicine is very appealing to our medical zeitgeist.

To best assess the value of measuring and fixing numbers in the elderly, we have only two tools: experience and scientific investigations. The former is a subjective means of assessment that doctors like myself utilize based on what years of practicing medicine have taught us, while the latter is alleged to be more objective and universally applicable. The truth is that most studies done on medications do not involve older people, as elderly patients typically are excluded from medication studies.[46] The studies that do have an older cohort rarely involve elderly participants on multiple medicines and with numerous medical problems reflective of the majority of older patients for whom I care. Also, most studies are sponsored by drug companies, and when the results of those studies verge from what the pharmaceuticals desire, the studies are not published.[47] [48] [49] [50] [51] Thus, when we assess the impact of disease and medication on older patients, we are using very little data that is reliable and meaningful.

When we do evaluate studies about numbers and the medicines used to treat those numbers, we must be aware of a very important nuance in the statistical presentation of data, something of which I have only recently become aware in my medical career. Most studies report their results in terms of **relative risk and benefit**. Those numbers could seem very impressive and make a test or treatment appear much more significant than it really is clinically. Contrarily, **absolute risk and benefit** is a much more revealing number, although rarely reported in the press or medical literature. In addition, it is important that the endpoint of a study reveals a **clinically significant** result. For instance, we do not care if a certain drug improves someone's number; we really care if the drug, by improving the number, helps them to be healthier or to live longer. Pharmaceutical companies that sell medicines and sponsor studies, medical researchers who gain prominence from demonstrating significant findings from their studies, and even members of the medical community who seek justification for aggressively labeling and treating disease, all rely on the allure of relative risk. A very small risk to a patient who has an abnormal number (such as high blood pressure), or a very small improvement in the patient's health from fixing that number, can be magnified into what seems to be a huge benefit when results are conveyed by relative risk and benefit rather than absolute risk and benefit. It is the latter, though, that is much more meaningful.

Consider that a lottery in this country has a huge payoff, and you learn that there is a fivefold higher chance of winning if you buy a ticket in Ohio instead of Maryland, where you live. Is it worth flying to Ohio to buy some tickets? The relative chance if winning in Ohio is five times higher, or 500 percent better, than if you purchase a ticket in Maryland, a very impressive number and perhaps worthy of a plane ticket. That is relative benefit. But the absolute benefit is much less impressive. If the chance of winning in Maryland is one out of ten million, and the chance of winning in Ohio is five out of ten million, then the absolute benefit of traveling to Ohio is a four out of ten million increased chance of winning, a much less appealing advantage. A five times relative benefit is really a four out of ten million absolute benefit. Thus, although in medical literature we hear almost extensively about the relative benefit and risk of certain medicines and treatments, that number typically will obscure the more relevant truth revealed by absolute risk and benefit.

It is important, then, to evaluate certain clinical situations where medicines are used to fix abnormal numbers in the elderly and to ascertain whether, in absolute terms, such interventions are justified. We also need to determine whether the risks of treating those numbers in the elderly are, in absolute terms, of concern to us. Medicare and the ACA, among other groups, are trying to assess and grade physician quality by tying it to the measurement and fixing of numbers and various medical conditions. This is being touted as a major thrust of reform: paying doctors for quality performance is perceived to be a revolutionary means of saving Medicare. But the validity of such an approach lays hidden in the numbers themselves. The question is: can we achieve improved health care outcomes in the elderly at a reduced cost by measuring and fixing numbers through models such as Medicare's quality indicators? The answer to that question reveals a very deeply rooted flaw in our geriatric health care delivery system, a flaw that has blinded many of those who are now trying to reform Medicare, and one that we will explore throughout this book.

## The Case of A-fib

*Medicare Quality Indicators state that all people over age 18 who are deemed to be high risk for stroke by specified criteria (*which include virtually all of the elderly) *should take Warfarin or a similar anticoagulant.*

The treatment of atrial fibrillation (A-fib) with Warfarin (Coumadin™) is a very good illustration of how relative risk can be a misleading means of evaluating a treatment. A-fib is a condition common in the elderly where the heart beats irregularly and rapidly. The primary difficulty with A-fib is that clots can accumulate in the heart and cause strokes.

To prevent this complication, doctors place patients on blood thinners such as Warfarin, an old rat poison that prevents clots from developing. In fact, the use of Warfarin in the elderly leads to a 50 percent reduction in strokes compared to the use of aspirin.[52] Because of such impressive results, virtually all doctors recommend the use of Warfarin in their older patients. Its use is standard of care and it is part of every clinical performance measure to which doctors are supposed to adhere. For most of my career, I never questioned its unassailable necessity; after all, why risk a stroke where is such an effective treatment available?

But numbers can be deceptive. Fifty percent reduction is a relative risk. In fact, the chance of an older person with A-fib getting a stroke is close to 6 percent a year. With aspirin that number moves down toward 4 percent. With Warfarin that number is closer to 2 percent.[53] True, Warfarin confers a 50 percent risk reduction compared to aspirin, but that is because it cuts the risk of stroke in half compared to aspirin, reducing it from 4.5 percent without any medicines to 2.5 percent with aspirin and to 1.4 percent with Warfarin.[54] Also, as many as half of the strokes that occur are minor and leave no lasting effects, so the clinically relevant improvement is half of those numbers, 1.25 percent risk with aspirin and 0.7 percent risk with Warfarin, or a 6/1000 decrease in the number of disabling strokes in people who take Warfarin instead of aspirin. That is the absolute risk reduction. Looking at it another way, there is a 99.3 percent chance of averting a clinically relevant stroke with Warfarin, and a 98.7 percent chance of averting a stroke with aspirin. When my patients hear about a 50 percent reduction in stroke, they are petrified about using aspirin instead of Warfarin, despite their fears of Warfarin. When I tell my patients about the absolute risk reduction, however, many of them prefer to take their chances and use aspirin, especially my patients who are older and are on many other medicines.

Why not just use Warfarin? Major strokes can be devastating, so even a small risk reduction can be significant. The problem is that Warfarin is not a benign drug. It interacts with virtually every medicine and food, from tea, to Tylenol, to a dinner salad. Patients must check their blood levels frequently; failure to do so could result in either ineffective doses or toxic doses. Patients on Warfarin bleed more, sometimes dangerously so, especially if they fall down, and especially if they are over eighty. **Studies suggest that the risk of serious bleeding ranges from 4–7 percent (40–70/1000) of patients each year**,[55] [56] which far exceeds the stroke reduction benefit of taking Warfarin in many cases. The risk of bleeding in the brain alone, which is another form of stroke (hemorrhagic stroke) is 0.6 percent (6/1000) higher in people taking Warfarin than those who take aspirin for A-fib,[57] meaning that almost the entire benefit of Warfarin in reducing stroke is erased by the increased risk of a brain bleed, both of which can similarly disable a patient.

For some patients, being on Warfarin is like having a leash around their necks; every illness they have, everything they put in their mouths, every medication change or new vitamin they take, every change in their behavior, every time they trip or bump their heads, every bruise or nosebleed, forces them to be aware of their Warfarin, to check their blood levels, and to talk to their doctors, to make adjustments in dose, or even to go to the hospital. To many of my patients, the stress of being on Warfarin is probably more likely to cause them a stroke than any risk reduction the drug may incur. And Warfarin itself can cause other problems directly, even an increase in the rate of osteoporotic fractures.[58] There are newer, more expensive drugs that have replaced Warfarin with similar risk reduction and without the need to check labs incessantly. But these too have side effects that are substantial, not the least of which is the inability to reverse the drug's effect for several days should a bleed occur. The use of anticoagulants such as Warfarin in A-fib demonstrates how people use relative risk to exaggerate the importance of employing certain aggressive interventions in older people even when the true efficacy is very small and the potential harm not insignificant. Still, every clinical guideline, including Medicare's quality indicators, assumes that Warfarin (or its equivalent) is an absolute necessity for eligible A-fib patients. Failure to use it is construed as a measure of poor quality care.

Warfarin is illustrative of our obsession with numbers and how that obsession in the elderly can be deleterious. Measuring Warfarin levels by blood provides a number called the INR. People on Warfarin are advised to maintain their INR within a narrow therapeutic window; if the number is too low they can have a stroke, and if it is too high they can bleed. Given that in many of my patients even a gust of wind seems to impact their INR, the fluctuations of INR are so wide that one cannot reliably know the value from day to day. However, my patients, or their families, are so focused on that number, so convinced that even a slight deviation from the norm will portend disaster, that they alter their lives dramatically to assure that the number remains good, often checking themselves more often than is required and refusing to eat foods they enjoy. Worse than that, many doctors who monitor their Warfarin are just as fixated on the number, and will do whatever is necessary to make sure that number stays within its narrow acceptable range, further adding to the stress that Warfarin inflicts on its users.

I have demented patients in nursing homes on Warfarin, elderly patients who fall, patients who cannot move or see, others who are on so many other medicines that their levels bounce everywhere. They will not stop this drug, so convinced are they that it is absolutely necessary to save them from a horrible stroke, a conviction reinforced by their doctors, their families, the lay press, and the deceiving relative risk improvement that the drug offers. The drug itself becomes a disease. No one seems to really care just how minimally Coumadin actually helps people stay healthy and how dangerous it can potentially be. They just care about the number. That has become the new marker of quality care.

## Hypertension

*Medicare Quality Indicators indicate that blood pressure should be kept below 140/90 in patients under the age of ninety.* (That number is expected to change to 150/90). *Any such patients diagnosed as having hypertension should be on an aspirin, be on a statin cholesterol medicine if*

*LDL cholesterol is elevated, have annual blood and urine kidney testing, have regular testing for diabetes, and should have their blood pressure treated.*

Blood pressure is another number that has reached a compulsive pitch among my elderly patients. Many are convinced that any bump in their pressure means that a stroke is imminent. Many of my patients check their pressure multiple times a day and make graphs and charts, trying to find patterns so they can ascertain methods of keeping the numbers normal. Those in nursing homes or who live with their family, who are having physical therapy or see another doctor, have their numbers checked often as well, frequently contacting me in distress that, even for a single reading, the number is dangerously high. And all of this is based on a number derived from a very imprecise blood pressure cuff that is user dependent and records a questionable pressure for a split second out of a person's life and extrapolates that number to have life-altering significance!

Very often my patients fall or are sick, are seen by a nurse, or are brought to the emergency room. During those moments their bodies and minds are stressed, and naturally their blood pressure is elevated. But no one seems to recognize the labile nature of pressure in the elderly; pressures can bounce haphazardly within a very wide range, soaring with a trauma as minor as the apprehension that occurs while the Velcro cuff expands on their arms. Blood pressure is so variablethat it can fluctuate 20 points just during one visit, especially when people get older; we know that there is a lack of correlation between a body's actual blood pressure and what we measure in the office.[59] [60]

After seeing a specialist or coming home from the hospital, many of my elderly patients emerge on more blood pressure medicines than they had going in. And very often, that is when they really start getting sick. The reality is that in the elderly I have seen much more illness caused by low pressure and the medicine used to treat hypertension than from high blood pressure itself, even though the parameters of normal pressure in the elderly are unknown and are probably higher than we think.

Simply equating a low blood pressure number to high-quality care, as quality indicators declare, obfuscates the importance in many old bodies of allowing the pressure to climb, at least some of the time. Once we shut off the body's blood pressure response by flooding it with medicines, we may be instigating a harmful cascade. I find it interesting that Medicare's quality indicators focus on preventing modestly high pressures, but say nothing about pushing pressures too low or side effects that occur with antihypertensive medicines.

Recently one of my patients saw a cardiologist, who constantly found her pressure to be very high. He put her on medicines, first one, then two, then five. The pressure did not drop, at least not while she was in his office. She admitted that when his nurse placed the cuff on her arm she became nervous, and that likely caused a spike in pressure. Now she lived in fear of stroke, taking her medicines religiously. But she could hardly stand up. She passed out several times, and became less able to walk. Even with physical therapy, her mobility declined, and she started to sleep more during the day. Her son bought her a blood pressure cuff and instructed her to check the pressure multiple times a day. Instead of attending activities, socializing, and exercising, this once strong woman now stayed in her apartment and took her blood pressure during the times she was not napping, reporting the numbers to her son, worrying about what would become of her. It took a lot of persuasion for me to convince her to drop her blood pressure medicines, especially since my advice contradicted that of the "expert" and of her son, but when she did stop them all, she reclaimed her life, becoming the active person she once was. She stopped checking pressure, and although she convinced herself that she was probably going to get a stroke from her decision, she believed that it was worth the benefit of feeling good.

But was she really going to get a stroke? When I was a medical student the SHEP study altered medical thinking by definitively proving that high systolic blood pressure in the elderly instigates strokes. Many since have criticized that study, showing that systolic blood pressure in the moderate-high range does not elevate stroke risk.[61] More significantly, recent studies have shown that in elders with heart disease, low blood pressure causes as many or more strokes as do high pressures.[62][63][64] A recent VA study looking at elderly men with kidney disease, many of whom also have diabetes, showed that lowering blood pressure below 130 led to increased death and no improvement in kidney function. As with studies that look at pressures in older people with strokes and heart attacks, this study found the optimal blood pressure to be 130–160,[65] which is far higher a number than most doctors or patients feel is acceptable.

Still, we in the medical world became obsessed with SHEP, and despite the very small absolute risk reduction of lowering blood pressure in our elderly patients, and despite the often debilitating side effects and interactions from pharmaceutical treatments, we push medicines and check more labs, as the quality indicators compel us to do. I have become more comfortable allowing pressures to run high in my older patients, especially if they feel better and function at a higher level with elevated pressures. Many of my patients are more energetic and cognitively alert at higher pressures, and many of my patients with poor balance fall less and walk better when their pressure medicines are reduced. Some of these patients are resistant to medicines; it is as if their bodies push up the pressure despite what we do to lower it. Likely their bodies are smarter than we are (and they have not read Medicare's quality indicators!). When doctors use medicine to reduce pressure below even 130, studies show that there is a potential for causing harm, including an increased death rate.[66][67][68] Some studies have shown that the withdrawal of blood pressure medicines typically cause no meaningful elevation of pressure or induction of cardiovascular disease in the majority of the elderly.[69][70] Recent articles published in many newspapers state that the parameters for ideal blood pressure in the elderly are too low, that in fact we should aim higher. This is a fact we have known for some time, but it is still not something that many doctors or patients believe, nor is it something that most quality indicators and clinical guidelines endorse. Given how unreliable our blood pressure measurements are, we are likely dropping people's pressures far lower than we even know.

More significantly, the drugs used to treat high blood pressure all have significant side effects and interactions that are accentuated as more drugs are tossed into an older body. Many of my patients are more tired, confused, and dizzy on their blood pressure medicine. Studies also have shown that low pressure can cause falls and fractures.[71] I have seen people hospitalized, incapacitated, and killed by these drugs. Still many of my patients, families, and doctors would rather obtain a perfect blood pressure number, despite what little that will do for the patient's actual health, rather than worry about how the drugs used to achieve that result may cause some minor "inconveniences" that incapacitate and maim them. Fixing the number has become a compulsion in our medical community, although it is an illusion built on the backs of our patients' health.

## Diabetes

*Medicare Quality Indicators state that in diabetics between 18–75 A1C should be maintained under 8, LDL cholesterol kept under 100, and blood pressure under 140/90. Presumably all these abnormal numbers are expected to be fixed with medicines. The guidelines also recommend periodic kidney and foot exams.*

Diabetes is another disease where the number is everything. People are frequently asking me to check their sugar, and often they do it on their own, multiple times a day, pricking their fingers to obtain a number that confers meaning to them, a number that if too high, even transiently, may portend devastating consequences. We are so obsessed with diabetes in our society that we have lowered the threshold of what it means to be diabetic, and have even invented a term called prediabetes to demonstrate that even slightly high blood sugars could be a sign of trouble ahead. We watch sugars closely, measure another number called A1C which gives us an average sugar over three months, and stress over whether we have achieved ideal diabetic control. Medicare's quality guidelines are somewhat forward thinking in not mandating tight control of diabetes in patients over the age of seventy-five, but they also do nothing to dissuade that practice. In fact Medicare pays for test strips, blood tests, and specialist visits for even the oldest diabetics, and does not comment on whether aggressively controlling sugars is efficacious for everyone. We as doctors are chided by the quality indicators for allowing sugars, cholesterol, and blood pressure to drift too high in diabetics under seventy-five, but we are not chastised for overtreating sugars with insulin and pills so that the number looks perfect all the time, especially in the very old, something that is frankly dangerous and potentially deadly. While treating diabetes in a sensible way makes sense, simply focusing on the numbers and applauding when they are very low can be clinically deceptive.

The reality is that in the elderly, there is scant evidence that maintaining tight control of blood sugars will confer any benefit at all. In fact, recent studies suggest just the opposite: controlling sugars strictly will actually trigger worse outcomes, including causing **more** death and **more** disability.[72][73][74][75][76] My own patients are adversely impacted when their sugars drop too low; not only can low sugar immediately kill them, but when they walk around with low sugars they are tired, dizzy, and more confused, much the same as occurs with my patients who have low blood pressure.[77][78] In nursing home eligible patients, in fact, a recent study showed improved function and fewer deaths in diabetics with the **worst** sugar control (A1C between eight and nine).[79] Like with many hypertensives, diabetics work diligently to normalize their numbers and push them as low as possible even though such aggressive number normalization exposes them to harm and to deterioration in quality of life. Still, following common lure and published guidelines, doctors, nurses, families, and my patients themselves check their sugars often with the stated goal of maintaining very low sugars. *The lower the better* seems to be the mantra in our diabetic universe. The number itself seems to obscure what aggressively fixing the number actually is doing to our patients.

Recently one of my patients, who is over ninety and living alone, although plagued by many chronic problems including pain, oxygen dependent lung disease, and poor balance, recently saw her endocrinologist. The diabetes doctor was not happy with her blood sugar control; her A1C had drifted over eight, and her twice a day sugar checks were sometimes close to 200 (although that occurred primarily after she ate). Although she was already on pills, the endocrinologist started insulin, persuading my patient that she had to start injecting herself with needles. My patient was very concerned about her sugars and believed that her life was in jeopardy if they remained elevated. Since she started the insulin her A1C came down to 7.3, although sugars occasionally dropped below eighty, something that make her happy, but frightened me. I explained that her preinsulin A1C was perfectly fine, and that she would gain no clinical ground by lowering it further; there would not be any reduction in stroke, heart attack, kidney disease, death, etc. If anything, she may hurt herself. But my patient was not moved by my reasoning. She wanted low numbers. Nothing else seemed to matter.

When I am evaluated by quality indicators, there is an assumption that I will use medicines to fix people's sugars when they drift too high. But how good are diabetic medicines? Certainly they are very effective at lowering sugars and A1C. If that were our endpoint of therapeutic success (as it is in the guidelines), then they would be wonderful treatments. But most of them have multiple interactions and side effects and, in some cases, have been shown to actually increase the chances of instigating a major medical event such as a heart attack and death.[80] [81] [82] [83] Still, even after knowing this, many of my patients or their caregivers would rather take medicines rather than allow their numbers to escalate beyond what they have been told is normal. Very often the families of my patients become the trigger of this behavior. Just today an older man with very mild dementia told me that his child calls him every morning to assure that dad checks his sugars. "I just make up numbers," the man said to me. "I give my son sugars that make him happy. I haven't really checked my sugars for months; I just throw out the supplies when they come. But I don't want him upset with me." Although the man believed he was being negligent, in fact he was taking a more prudent path than his son, or society, encouraged of him. He felt well, he was not stressed by his numbers, and likely he would live longer and better than had he been more diligent with his glucose control. He may have failed Medicare's quality indicators, but he was receiving quality care.

# Cholesterol

*Medicare Quality Indicators look at the need to check and reduce LDL cholesterol in certain conditions such as hypertension, diabetes, and coronary artery disease. They use LDL of 100 above which is abnormal, but do not comment of how to treat.*

Number fixation is perhaps most evident in the realm of cholesterol. I have had patients who simply want to know their cholesterol so they can talk about it at dinner with their friends. I have families who fear taking their mom or dad off cholesterol medicine even though they are demented in a nursing home, so fearful are they that the cholesterol number will worsen off the medicines. Cholesterol is easy to measure, is in the news, and has entered our common lore as being a marker of how healthy we are. By fixing cholesterol we are cheating death.

One of my patients came to me on two cholesterol medicines and a few supplements that also control cholesterol. Looking through his records I could find no good diagnoses that would support such aggressive treatment (no heart disease, no strokes, etc.), and his last cholesterol check was perfect. I advised him to eliminate one of his medicines, Zetia, which has been shown to lower the cholesterol numbers without necessarily lowering rates of heart attacks or strokes.[84] He reluctantly agreed, but several months later, when he asked me to recheck his cholesterol, his numbers had gone up. He became very nervous.

"These labs are not good," he said to me. "I don't want to walk around with those cholesterol levels."

"But," I tried to reassure him, "the numbers may not be perfect, but they are OK. And stopping the Zetia hasn't increased your risk of getting any illness. You are just on one less medicine, that's all."

He accepted my explanation, for a day or two. But the next week he called my office and asked for a refill of his Zetia. He simply could not bear to live with the higher numbers, even if fixing those numbers did nothing to improve his chance of living better or longer. The illusion of perfect numbers was more important to him than the reality of what those numbers really meant.

There is great controversy about whether any treatment of cholesterol in the elderly is warranted.[85] [86] Statins have been shown to help people with heart disease and strokes, but recent evidence has shown minimal clinically significant benefit in elderly people without risk factors.[87] [88] [89] [90] Even the studies that claim some improvement in outcome among selected elders on statins show a tiny absolute risk reduction usually measured in days of life saved. Cholesterol medicines have significant side effects in the elderly, especially muscle weakness and pain, and do have interactions with other medicines. They can impair quality of life and they add another element of stress to an older person's already stressful life.

Once can argue, despite the conflicting evidence, that after a stroke or heart attack, or even in patients at high risk for such events, statin drugs are potentially efficacious if patients have a reasonably long life expectancy. But that is true despite their cholesterol number. The fact that Zetia can drop the cholesterol number as much as a statin, but that only the latter actually meaningfully reduces reoccurrence of stroke or heart attack in certain people, implies that the number alone is not what is really important. Many doctors try to push that number as low as possible by adding more and more medicines, believing that the number itself has singular significance; up until recently they were supported by clinical guidelines that compelled them to view LDL as a marker of a disease. Interestingly, new guidelines actually dissuade doctors from reducing LDL to a predefined target value.[91] That is a breath of fresh air in our number-obsessed medical world; the guidelines actually suggest the use of statins in specific clinical situations where patients may benefit, regardless of their cholesterol numbers, and with attention paid to their age. Unfortunately, cholesterol guidelines, as with hypertension where prior guidelines encouraged lower target blood pressures and diabetes where prior guidelines encouraged higher target sugars, shift with the time, and thus if we follow today's guidelines, we may be out of compliance with tomorrow's. Cholesterol is just a number. Patients are much more complicated than numbers.

## Osteoporosis and More

*Medicare Quality Indicators suggest that all people over the age of sixty-five should be screened for osteoporosis by bone density testing, and that people over the age of fifty with known osteoporosis should be prescribed medicines for their condition.*

So many of our treatments and guidelines are based on negligible absolute risk reduction and poor data that are not applicable to most elderly patients, while inducing side effect and interaction profiles that put old patients at risk for functional decline, impaired quality of life, and serious medical complications. A salient example includes osteoporosis medicines like Alendronate (Fosamax) that can improve poor bone density numbers (T values) when evaluated by bone densitometry testing, but that may have marginal to negligible absolute benefit on fracture risk, which is a much more clinically relevant endpoint. While studies tout a 55 percent relative reduction of hip fracture risk for women who use bisphosphonates like Alendronate, the absolute risk reduction is much smaller, such that for every thousand women in the high osteoporotic risk group who take Alendronate, approximately two will have hip fractures prevented. While the drugs do seem to have more efficacy in preventing spine fractures, those fractures are often found on x-rays but do not cause any pain, and thus are not clinically significant.[92 93 94 95]

Certainly there is little or no evidence that Alendronate helps prevent hip fractures in lower-risk women without prior fracture and has a negligible impact on spine fracture in this group.[96] Bisphosphonates also have multiple common side effects, such as increased bone pain and worse acid reflux. Recent studies suggest that long-term use of Alendronate can actually cause increased risk of spontaneous fractures, causing some to advocate limiting their use to five years.[97] Thus we can fix numbers with bisphosphonates, we can demonstrate impressive relative risk improvements, but in fact the drug will help two high-risk women prevent fractures in a year for every thousand women who must take it on a regular basis and expose themselves to drug interactions and medical risk. It can also increase fracture risk with long-term use. Measuring and fixing a bone density number has nebulous clinical value.

Measuring and tightly controlling thyroid disease, anemia, testosterone deficiency, kidney failure, and various other abnormal numbers that can be discovered through tests and "improved" by medicine can be similarly ineffective if not harmful. Mild thyroid disease, for example, rarely causes meaningful clinical improvement when treated with replacement, and yet such treatment and number fixing is considered the standard of care in geriatrics. Anemia is common in the elderly, frequently looked for by a blood test, sometimes treated (typically with iron, which can constipate people), but rarely does treatment lead to clinically meaningful outcomes unless the condition is severe. We are told to measure and fix vitamin levels, monitor kidney and liver function regularly, check urine for blood and protein, check heights and weights and pressures at every visit; so many numbers translate to so many diagnoses that lead to so many medicines, with so little evidence that our deluge of probing and treating is truly helping our older patients to live longer and better. And when you add up all the medicines that one of my patients may require to repair all of his aberrant numbers, the side effects and interactions multiply. The medical community's fixation on numbers, and the recent push to equate number fixing with quality care, has become more important than the reality of what the medicines used to treat those numbers may be actually doing to the patients forced to swallow them.

## Treating Annoying Problems in the Aged

On September 11th 2001, at 9:00 a.m. Mrs. M. walked into my office for her appointment. She had a litany of complaints to share with me, and so she whipped out her two-page list.

My memories of 9/11 are infused with Mrs. M.'s visit. It seemed interminable. Between items on her list that ranged from sore toes to bad breath, heads started popping into my exam room door relaying small slices of information that were both shocking and unbelievable— a single-engine plane hit the World Trade tower, no it turns out it was a commercial jet, the second tower was hit, the Pentagon was hit—and I jolted out of the room and ran down the hall to watch with so many other silent bodies the events that were to transform our world.

"Sorry about that," I would say after every excursion to the TV as I popped back in to the visit with Mrs. M. "It looks like there is a full-scale terrorist attack against us."

"Really?" she said. "That is too bad. Well, going down, number thirteen, I have a small growth on my back I want you to look at."

So it proceeded for an eternal stretch of agony.

From that day on, Mrs. M. became Mrs. 9/11. I joked with her about it for many years. She always shook her head, embarrassed, claiming that she had not realized what was transpiring that day until she returned to her apartment and turned on the TV. So intent was she in dissecting her list that nothing beyond its twenty-plus issues penetrated her thoughts.

The list is everything to many of my patients. It is imperative at every visit that they recite its contents and that I acknowledge the severity of every one of its items. It took me years of practice to realize that patients like Mrs. 9/11 never expect me to resolve their listed woes, but rather to simply empathize with and recognize the manifestations of aging. Every item on her list, every problem that comes with aging, can be analyzed, tested, and treated. For every ailment there is a test, a medicine, a cure.

With aging comes not only disease but also disability. Nuisance problems crop up like weeds, and often they can impair a person's ability to function independently. From fatigue, to urinary incontinence, to constipation, to various types of pain, aging is not without its challenges. Most elderly people have two choices for how to confront nuisance: try to extirpate it, or try to deal with it. The latter is accomplished by means of accommodation and acclimation, and is the recipe for successful aging. The former leads to stress, adverse consequences, tests, excessive medicine use, frustration, and often increased disability.

Many drugs exist that erase the ravages of aging, most of them cluttered with potential side effects, few of them able to produce anything but marginal absolute risk reduction. There are incontinence drugs like Ditropan and Detrol, GERD medicines like Nexium and Protonix, ED medicines like Viagra and Cialis. There is no better way to confront nuisance than with medicines, and for every problem an elderly person can develop there is a drug to fix it. TV ads are cluttered with grateful people having been cured of their enlarged prostates, their incontinence, their erectile dysfunction, their pain. I have never seen such happy people as those who live in the world of TV drug ads. Drug ads cannot tell lies, but they can show only people who improve dramatically, cite only the studies that support them, tell us only the good that is achieved (other than the quickly mumbled list of side effects at the end of every ad that we have become conditioned to ignore).

Americans take more medicines than anyone else in the world without better outcomes and typically without life-preserving or life-improving results.[98] Those of us who practice geriatric medicine fight every day to get people off their long list of medicines touted to cure practically everything and to be absolutely essential to their health and well-being. It is a battle against a powerful message, one that promises that aging itself can be cured. It is a battle against many deep-seated perceptions, underscored by the quality indicators with which Medicare will now be judging us. When we do win, we almost always see satisfying results. But when we lose, we watch our patients dwindle, still convinced that all of their fifteen drugs and supplements are necessary, still happy about the thoroughness of their care, but still unable to dance in the woods like those people on the TV commercials.

# Dementia

*Medicare Quality Indicators recommend various tests for dementia that allow the disease to be characterized and staged, as well as various forms of screening and counseling, but do not comment on the use of medication in its treatment.*

Dementia is perhaps the most devastating illness for which patients and families seek a miracle solution. While some of the elderly simply become forgetful, an outcome that is expected as people age, others lapse into true dementia, where function declines and the brain's capacity to reason collapses. Several drugs have been touted to improve dementia, especially Alzheimer's disease, from Aricept, to Exelon, to Namenda. But again, despite curves and graphs that demonstrate the remarkable relative risk reduction of disease progression from these drugs, the absolute clinical improvement is negligible for most patients, while the studies themselves may be unreliable.[99]

No drugs actually alter the course of dementia; at best they help symptoms. Improvement in clinical trials is measured by numbers; patients take a test, typically scored on a scale of 70, and if they improve their score by 4 points or more then the drug is believed to be effective. It is unclear how much these research-derived numerical scales actually translate to clinically relevant change. In fact studies that measure functional improvement that is recognized by their caregivers are less convincing. Most of the time numerical improvement, even with these scales, has been small, and the dropout rate of patients from the studies due to side effects has been very high.[100] [101] [102] Also, none of the studies extend beyond a year in duration, and the improvement that is seen seems to level off after about 4–6 months, after which drug efficacy parallels placebo.[103] So it is unclear just how long the very modest effect of these drugs will persist. Studies have shown that approximately 9–30 percent of people with dementia who take these drugs have some symptomatic improvement compared to placebo.[104] But interestingly, approximately 30 percent of demented people have a response to placebo, showing that there is a very large placebo effect to treatment.[105] Namenda, a newer and more expensive drug, has even less evidence to back its use.[106] [107] [108] Also, no study has demonstrated that any one drug is better than another, or that a combination of these drugs is better than a single drug alone.[109] Again, even those who do have a response often have a clinically marginal change for a very brief duration; typically they merely demonstrate a transient improvement in their memory-score numbers.

On the drugs or off, people with dementia decline, they become disabled and nonfunctioning, and many eventually require twenty-four-hour care or admission to long-term care facilities. The drugs offer an illusory hope that this terrible disease can somehow be stopped in its tracks. Often they are used as a crutch, while other more proven methods of helping people with dementia are neglected, such as socialization and exercise.[110] [111] [112] [113] The drugs also have substantial side effects. About 10 percent of people on these drugs have significant gastrointestinal side effects that force them to stop the medicines,[114] and a small but measurable number have very serious side effects such as complete heart block, fainting, and hip fractures.[115] Medicare B pays for tests and specialty visits; Medicare D pays for the drugs. No part of Medicare will help demented patients or their families pay for day care, home care, exercise programs, or other proven methods of helping them cope with the disease.

Pharmaceutical representatives who have talked to me claim that not only do these drugs help slow the progression of Alzheimer's disease in a significant way (and they have skewed graphs to prove it), but also that if the drug is stopped the patient will lose everything he or she has gained from the drug and will never recover. Such scare tactics convince doctor and patient alike that not using this miracle of science is irresponsible and cruel, and stopping the drug is even worse. Many neurologists and psychologists with whom I work convince patients and families that these drugs are both necessary and effective. Quality indicators and clinical guidelines encourage doctors to treat dementia, and the treatments most available and accepted are these drugs. Such drugs are just another example of how we have all been convinced that aggressive treatment can cure the worst ravages of aging by fixing nebulous numbers, even if such lore verges far from the truth and can actually be harmful and deceptive.

## Drug Advertising

Pharmaceutical companies, often much maligned by those who seek to reform our health care industry, benefit greatly by our quest to repair numbers and symptoms of aging with medicines. The clinical studies that they sponsor report dramatic medication impact almost exclusively in relative risk/benefit language. That language is then picked up by the press, which reports it to the public. We hear frequently about 50 percent risk reduction, 20 percent improvement, and other often deceiving figures that obscure whether a drug is truly beneficial. The risks of drugs are typically glossed over. In addition, pharmaceutical companies advertise directly to the public, using doctor and patient actors to demonstrate medication wonderment. But perhaps most concerning is how such companies market their drugs to the health care delivery industry, coaxing doctors and other professionals to believe that the answer to much of aging's decline lays in a bottle of pills.

Many studies have explored the intoxicating impact of drug advertising,[116][117] and I do not plan to comment extensively on that reality other than saying that many of my elderly patients, and their families, believe that medicines can repair much of what is going wrong with aging due to what they have seen or read in ads. Drug companies have a right to advertise and try to sell their products. They send representatives into doctor's offices, they disseminate their word directly to consumers, and they compete with each other for a voracious market. It is not their actions that are most disturbing. It is rather the fact that doctors and patients alike buy into their message. It is that the lay press publishes their dogma, using relative risk to demonstrate a drug's magical properties without exploring whether the drug really is clinically efficacious. It is that few even in academic medicine try to counter the myths. The impact of pharmaceutical companies on the medical community is well documented,[118] [119] [120] and I am no less immune to its power than any others.

During my early days as a doctor I appreciated an occasional foray into Baltimore for a good meal, sometimes at Ruth's Chris, sometimes at another restaurant that sat well above my price range of possibilities. Our local drug reps were always happy to accommodate. They invited us out quite frequently, sometimes to restaurants, sometimes to Orioles games, sometimes even on trips. A few of us from work would accept and go as a group. There we would start with an open bar and a bowl of jumbo shrimp, then a brief talk by a doctor paid by the drug company to say something nice about a particular drug within the guise of an unbiased scientific talk, then we would have our full meal with steak and potatoes and dessert. It was something to which I looked forward and to which I became almost addicted after a while. I saw nothing wrong with it. But then one day, after a very mediocre drug dinner at the newly opened (and now extinct) ESPN zone, the drug rep who sponsored the dinner walked into my office and, in front of patients, handed me a trophy as a gesture of thanks for using his drug. To me that was a wake-up call, and my taste for pharmaceutical-sponsored dinners abruptly ended.

While a resident at the University of Virginia, where the faculty looked down on drug reps and attempted to keep them out of the institution (even while many of them were being paid by drug companies either to do research or to give talks, something endemic in the world of academic medicine),[121] we welcomed the reps because they provided us with something much deserved. Residency was difficult, to say the least, and we were paid very little to work like dogs. The drug reps offered us a package of perks and a few slaps on the back. My favorite rep sold nicotine patches, which at the time were prescription drugs. He financed a program that I ran to help patients and employees quit smoking, providing me with free patches to give to my class participants. He twice sent me and twenty other residents on an amazing weekend adventure to the New River Gorge in West Virginia for a white water rafting trip. When I left residency he offered to fly me and my family to Lake Tahoe to participate in a smoking cessation workshop, where we would be wined and dined for a week. He was always good to me, and never seemingly asked for anything in return. Throughout residency various reps provided us with weekly lunches, meals at good Charlottesville restaurants, and even trips to local resorts. In fact, my drug company perks constituted some of the best memories of those three years. Such extravagance is no longer permitted, although one can still find a good lunch or dinner gratis if one looks around any medical corner.

Some drug reps are true salesmen, such as the man who gave me a trophy, but most whom I have encountered genuinely believe in their drugs and want to convince us to share in that belief. They do not force us to use any particular medicine. It is our choice what we actually prescribe. Sometimes patients request drugs that they have seen advertised, sometimes doctors prescribe drugs that drug reps convince them are effective; almost always Medicare D will pay for those choices. But wrapped around every decision to use a medicine is a deep-seated contention that medicines can cure virtually everything, and that newer medicines are even more effective than their predecessors. And the language of all pharmaceutical reps with whom I have had contact is that of relative risk.

One troubling behavior practiced by pharmaceutical companies is to make sure that their reps fill doctors' closets with free samples of all the newest and most expensive medicines. In my current practice, where I have established no ties with drug companies and thus have no pens, lunches, or samples, I cannot offer any free boxed medicines to my patients, and several patients have even thought about leaving me because of that. They have become very dependent on the samples, especially when it comes to expensive medicines. Those who have good insurance start with the samples and then buy the medicines, the precise formula that the drug companies count on.[122] If a patient develops a new diagnosis, we will often first try a drug that is in our sample closet. We can give them a couple of weeks of the drug, and if it works then we can give them a prescription. But the drugs in the closet are the most expensive and least-tested ones on the market. Once our patients become accustomed to those drugs, they will either need to pay for the medicine, have their insurance pay for it, or become dependent on a supply of samples. Either way, they are now taking a new, expensive medicine while an older, more tested medicine could have been given in its stead, or perhaps no medicine at all. Now that I have no samples filling my closet, I almost always start my patients on old, cheap generic medicines if they even need medical treatment. There are a ton of them for every condition, and they have been well tested over the years both in terms of safety and efficacy.

During one of President Obama's town meetings to promote his Affordable Care Act, a member of the audience who supported health care reform said indignantly that his insurance company had tried to switch him from brand-named Lipitor to generic simvastatin, and that his heart doctor wanted him on Lipitor, and how would the President's plan prevent such an outrage. I was curious to see how President Obama would respond. In fact, he tried to explain that often a less expensive generic like simvastatin is equally effective and should be the preferred drug. But his statement, which was bravely accurate, seemed to soar over the head of the man, who continued to complain about having to take generics. There are generics for virtually every major drug class that work just as well (or equally not as well, as the case may be) as the more expensive drugs. But no one promotes the generics. No generic drug makers give doctors lunches, provide samples, or flood the market with ads to push their drugs. Prilosec (Omeprazole) when it came out revolutionized treatment of acid reflux. They called it the purple pill and we were barraged by advertising touting its revolutionary benefits. But when its patent expired, the parent drug company of Omeprazole invented Nexium, the new purple pill. Omeprazole changed it color and became relegated as a cheap ineffective generic, while Nexium was the new miracle drug. The ploy worked. Nexium supplanted Prilosec in the hearts and minds of American consumers. Omeprazole became just another over-the-counter medicine. Both Omeprazole and Nexium are similarly efficacious and with identical side effects.[123]

In my recent career I have found that many of the products most heavily advertised by pharmaceutical companies are copycat drugs, something borne out by the literature.[124] These are drugs that do not have a novel purpose, but rather tweak an existing drug to give it a new patent and a more expensive price tag. Then the company's scientists work hard to prove that the new drug is somehow superior to the virtually identical medicines already on the market; they bend some curves and exaggerate some relative risk numbers, and then at least for a few years they feed their reps with enough ammo to peddle the drugs to hungry doctors and consumers.

The point is that we already have too many drugs on the market that are of questionable efficacy. These can include "cures" for urinary incontinence, depression, and acid reflux, to name a few. Do incontinence medicines really work? Probably not, but they all can cause their patients to have dry mouth, constipation, more falls, and worse confusion. Acid reflux medicines, while often able to relieve symptoms of heart burn, can increase the risk of bone fractures while providing questionable long-term efficacy. We use many depression medicines to "cure" fatigue and boredom, common problems in the elderly better treated with socialization and exercise, free of the very real side effects most depression medicines deliver.[125] [126] [127] We treat toe nail fungus, arthritis, dizziness, poor appetite, drippy noses, constipation, and so many other common ailments in our aging patients with drugs that are nominally effective, interact with other medicines, and all have a laundry list of side effects that frequently occur. Drugs cannot cure the ravages of aging. Usually they just get in the way.

# Supplements

As a side note, I should state that supplements and vitamins are not necessarily any better than prescription pills. They also have side effects and interactions and, unlike medicines, most are not regulated by the FDA nor are they well studied. Two miracle drugs that were evaluated for their curative powers in heart disease were folic acid and vitamin E. Both, after they were subjected to good double-blind placebo studies, and despite theoretical promise for their worth, were found to be ineffective and perhaps harmful.[128] [129] [130] [131] A more recent study of vitamin E did show some benefit in people with dementia,[132] but the research on memory supplements is very fickle, and a positive study is often followed by a negative one, leaving doctor and patient often in a quandary. Also, the improvements are typically clinically of minimal significance. People with memory loss also reach for coconut oil and ginseng, despite a complete lack of evidence that any of these or so many other products accomplish anything of value.[133] Calcium supplementation, which is recommended for older people and is widely taken by my patients, has never been demonstrated to definitively reduce fracture rates in older people, and potentially can increase the risk of heart attacks and other untoward effects.[134] [135] [136] [137] [138] [139]Fish oil, which is also popular among my patients, has not been demonstrated to reduce heart disease, and may have significant side effects such as increasing cancer risk.[140] [141] [142] [143] Aspirin,[144] multiple vitamins, and anti-oxidants[145] [146] [147] [148] [149] [150] [151]all have been promoted to succor the ravages of aging, but the reality verges far from perception, and these supplements are often either ineffective or actually harmful. In fact, even more than with pharmaceuticals, supplements can promise the world and deliver nothing, as they are not subject to any rigorous FDA standards. In addition they interact with other medicines and add to a patient's expansive medicine burden within his/

her body. Now we hold vitamin D up as a new savior, with a few small studies touted to support its wonderment. Perhaps it will prove to be of use, perhaps not, but certainly it will not reverse the nuisances and disability that aging inevitably instigates.

One cannot discount the impact of persuasion on the perceived value of a drug or supplement. When friends and doctors and advertisements and TV shows pound into someone's head that a drug is good, then often that person will believe that it is working, even if it does nothing at all. Such a phenomenon is called the placebo effect.[152] A recent study examined the power of placebos when patients with upper respiratory infections received either placebo or an herb called Echinacea. Those who believed that Echinacea works to help colds, and those who thought they were receiving the herb, regardless of whether they received the open label medicine or a placebo, had a significantly shorter duration of their cold and a less severe cold. Their belief in the herb's power caused them to have clinical improvement.[153]

With many of our drugs and supplements, the placebo effect may be the most potent benefit patients will receive. As an intern at the University of Virginia Hospital I worked under a resident who was a bit odd. He could not tolerate patients who came in with complaints of vague pain and then demanded narcotics, many of whom were admitted to the hospital every week. One night he assembled us and a few willing nurses to take care of an infamous frequent flier pain medication seeker. He told the patient that he had access to a new drug, Norsaline, which was stronger than any other pain reliever available. However, the drug could play havoc on the body, and it needed to be monitored closely. Would the patient want to try it? The patient, who was writhing in pain, agreed. We put him a room and hooked him up to an IV, as several nurses monitored his vital signs. Then the resident started the Norsaline drip, which was in fact a bag of normal saline, or salt water. Nurses shouted out vital signs with consternation, the resident changed the rate of flow, chaos consumed the room. After the bag finished the patient smiled, saying that he never felt better in his life.

That is the power of placebo, an impact imparted by so many of our drugs and supplements, and by so much of our medical delivery system. Normal saline of course was safe, even if the ethics of the resident's actions could be questioned. But many of the other drugs we shove into our elderly patients' guts are not so blessed with innocuity, even if they often do offer a very valuable placebo benefit. If it were not for the litany of side effects and interactions that such drugs induce, then perhaps such faith would be sufficient justification for their use. But given the harsh impact of drugs on the elderly, and the costs of such treatment, our promotion of drugs as an answer to aging's woes is a dangerous seed to plant.

## Clinical Guidelines

We have talked about clinical guidelines largely in the context of Medicare's Quality Indicators. Clinical guidelines are consensus statements drafted by "experts" in a particular field largely based on the conclusions of prevailing medical literature. They are typically extremely generic; it is rare that guidelines are applicable to elderly patients whose multiple illnesses, medicines, expectations, susceptibility to side effects, and life expectancy make each older person unique and not able to be squeezed into the rigid mold of a guideline. Also, as discussed, many studies used to script guidelines are sponsored by pharmaceutical companies and evaluate very few elderly subjects. And many of their "expert" authors have questionable motives, a very specialized agenda, and a minimal understanding of the aging process.[154] A recent *Annals of Internal Medicine* editorial suggested that clinical guidelines do have some validity, but while primary care doctors like me disdain the highly interventional guidelines scripted by specialists, the specialists similarly scoff at the anti-interventional guidelines developed in the academic primary care community. All guidelines, the author suggests, are so sensationalized by the press so as to obscure their real value.[155] Guidelines also will fluctuate based on which group pens them, and in what year they are penned. Some guidelines from the last decade would be considered substandard medical care today. If we are going to place clinical guidelines on a pedestal and label them as effective tools upon which to base quality medical care, then we have to admit that many doctors have and continue to practice poor medical care by adhering to guidelines that have been discredited, and that perhaps the doctors of tomorrow will disparage us for adhering to the soon-to-be discredited guidelines of today.

Medicare's quality indicators are fairly basic guidelines with some flexibility built into them. Many are based on the US Preventive Services Task Force (USPSTF) guidelines that tend to be very conservative in their recommendations. But the quality indicators stress when to test and treat, rather than when not to. They are also far too generic to be relevant to many of the older patients upon whom we are being instructed to use them. And to many of us in primary care, quality indicators force us to devote too much of our effort to documenting how often we order certain tests, fix certain numbers, and use certain medicines by employing a tightly scripted format that is time-consuming and not constructive.

In some larger health plans physicians are judged by specific clinical guidelines, many of which encourage them to fix the very numbers that we have demonstrated have little relevance to the elderly, such as tight control of hypertension and diabetes, and the use of statins in patients with high cholesterol.[156] Two of the primary innovations of Medicare reform and the ACA, the development of Accountable Care Organizations (ACOs) and of quality indicators called PQRS (both of which we will talk about in more detail later) presume that patient outcome can be improved by adherence to specified clinical guidelines, and that such adherence can be used to define a physician's performance. In the Northern Maryland ACO to which I have been assigned, I will be judged by how well I control sugars, blood pressure, and cholesterol and how often I prescribe specific types of drugs that are deemed to be efficacious in conditions such as congestive heart failure and coronary artery disease. [157] Clinical guidelines are becoming a vital instrument used to drive health care reform; gradually a larger part of our Medicare payment is becoming contingent on our compliance with the quality indicators. Pay for performance is being touted as an effective way to cut costs and improve quality.

But how effective are mandated performance measures that are scripted from clinical guidelines in achieving these goals? It is hard to imagine how asking us to fill out complicated forms indicating how we measure, record, and treat specific ailments and numbers in our elderly patients will save Medicare money. If anything it will lead to more tests, more referrals, more medication use, and more side effects, all at a higher cost. The process of completing ACO and PQRS quality measurement forms, on top of several other "Medicare innovations" that are measuring the "quality" of our care (including Wellness notes and Meaningful Use requirements, which we will discuss later as well) is laborious and expensive, and takes away time from quality patient care. By dictating what we should be discussing with our patients, and by specifically telling us how to have that conversation, quality indicators directly infringe upon the doctor-patient relationship. Geriatric medicine is a much more nuanced field than can be measured by preordained quality indicators. My eighty-five-year-old patient in a nursing home, and my eighty-five-year-old patient who came off the golf course, each has a different set of values, problems, and needs that will impact how he perceives a certain test or intervention. A meaningful discussion between a patient and doctor will lead to a meaningful resolution. None of this can be accomplished within the narrow scope of quality indicators.

Clinical guidelines, by advocating number chasing and treatment, also can lead to polypharmacy, a true danger in the geriatric population. Currently I am recertifying for the Internal Medicine Boards and am taking a home study course to get me ready. The tapes to which I am listening, fifty hours in all, are copied from a Board Review course taught by physicians from a major medical center. These people are academics and specialists, picked as being experts in their field, similar to the people who write clinical guidelines and orchestrate Medicare reform. What is most amazing to me is what each of them perceives to be the standard of care in terms of medicine use. The cardiologists would have the vast majority of my elderly patients on 5–10 drugs depending on their conditions, the osteoporosis expert wants at least three drugs and vitamins, the renal doctor is expecting a few drugs and vitamins, the ophthalmologist a few vitamins, and every other specialist a few more drugs, each one absolutely necessary for the survival of that particular specialist's organ of interest. They all demand fairly regular lab testing and number monitoring. What one specialist considers standard of care for a certain aliment another specialist bashes as being harmful to another ailment that is likely to coexist with the first. During the Internal Medicine Boards Review course one of the cardiologists told us that in congestive heart failure (CHF), a condition that occurs when the heart is not able to capably pump all of its contents to the body, it was standard of care to use certain drugs to adequately treat the condition. Medicare's quality indicators list some, but not all, of the drugs she deemed essential. But then the cardiologist said something both illuminating and frightening. She said that sometimes these essential drugs can cause the blood pressure to drop too low. Don't worry about it, she callously stated. Even if the pressure drops too low, the drugs will still do their job. You just have to be tough and hold your ground.

And that is another flaw of clinical guidelines that evaluate one number or disease in isolation from the rest of a person's mind and body. We as geriatricians know that when the blood pressure is too low our older patients are tired, they fall down and break bones, they are dizzy, and they feel lousy. Maybe they even become sicker and die like the Virginia farmer I treated. So is it really worth it to be on a preordained assortment of drugs and to fix a predefined set of numbers, with perhaps a tiny absolute risk reduction, if the consequences can be functionally disastrous and the outcome not meaningfully improved? And what if the patients are on other drugs for other conditions that interfere with these drugs, or what if these drugs make other conditions they have worse? What is the proof that the four essential drugs for congestive heart failure genuinely help an eighty-five-year-old woman with poor balance, chronic back pain, memory loss, and dizziness who is on eight other medicines? Have studies been conducted that prove efficacy for that patient? The answer is no. The answer is that clinical guidelines, and the vast majority of studies, do not apply to most Medicare patients.

It is important to understand that there is ample evidence that the more drugs you pile into a person's body, the less effective and more dangerous each drug is, especially as people age.[158] [159] [160] [161] Some have said that when a person is on more than six drugs (including supplements) then the side effects of each one doubles. And some data suggest that up to 400,000 people are killed or maimed every year by adverse drug reactions.[162] So although each and every drug seems to be necessary to erase and reduce disease burden, fix a number, or improve a nuisance, the combination of all of them can tear an elderly body to shreds. Thus when clinical guidelines push us to measure and fix more numbers, when each number and each nuisance demands more and more drugs for its resolution, a body that sits in a very delicate balance between function and disarray gets pushed closer to the latter. All of us who practice geriatrics see this happen. But as geriatric doctors, our "performance" will now be measured by our ability to "fix" numbers and flood our patients with even more poison. This is touted as Medicare reform!

Quality indicators, and our fixation with number measurement and number fixing through medicines, has led us down a very precarious road. Once we believe that an older person's health status can be equated to a number, and once we convince ourselves that by fixing that number with medicines we are fixing the patient, then we are led to believe that the ravages of aging can be systematically assaulted. Aging itself can fall prey to medical science as long as we probe and treat aggressively enough. This is what I label as thorough medical care. Very often my patients, or their families, laud *thorough* doctors who are monitoring their kidney function, or fixing their diabetes, or keeping a tight watch on their heart. Thorough medicine is not necessarily effective medicine;

for elderly patients it often causes more harm than good; it raises expectations beyond what is reasonable for doctor and patient alike, and its huge price tag is largely financed by Medicare. But once the idea percolates that aging can be reversed, then a cascade of interventions are possible, each more expensive and potentially dangerous than the next. And so we move down a road of aggressive care, a road flooded with pills of every color and shape, tests of every form, treatments of every type. In a world of common sense, people age, and that is OK. Problems occur that are not amenable to simple fixes, and that is OK, too. We should accept that, and try to promote happiness and activity as age chips away at our patients. We should utilize tests and treatments judiciously, realizing that too much of anything is potentially harmful and that what works for one patient many not work for all. And we should be realistic about the fact that excessive treatment may lead to excessive decline. But in our world as it exists today, number-chasing and medication obsession are the first ingredients of "thorough" medical care, the dangerous philosophy we will explore throughout the book.

# 2

# DEFINING THOROUGH: FINDING AND FIXING EVERYTHING

*Medicare is like a buffet of health care. For a very small
price you can eat all that you want, and are encouraged to do so,
but in the end, instead of feeling better you just get sick.*

Americans perceive that our current high-tech medical system is the best in the world, despite dubious evidence to support that claim.[163] [164] From MRIs to cardiac stress tests, from mammograms to colonoscopies, from full blood tests to full exams, we as doctors have at our disposal multiple tools to get inside our patients' bodies and search for trouble.

Technology in health care has skyrocketed in this country. Both doctors and patients are enamored of technology,[165] believing that tests and procedures help eradicate disease and extend life. The use of radiologic imaging in particular is accelerating rapidly without any evidence that x-rays and scans are extending or improving health for the population as a whole.[166] Since the early 1990s the ordering of head CT scans has doubled, chest CT scans have quintupled, head MRIs quadrupled, spine MRIs have increased six fold, and hip and knee MRIs have increased tenfold.[167] The same is true of procedures that are touted as lifesaving and that are similarly skyrocketing in their frequency of being performed, despite specious evidence. Says one author who has studied medical care: "Many doctors are happy to embrace the data that confirm their preconceived notions about the effectiveness of invasive treatment, while ignoring studies that don't."[168]

But our oldest patients are littered with disease, much of it hidden beneath a thin veil of accommodation. If we look hard enough, we will likely uncover medical conditions that may be well compensated and we may uncover medical conditions that will never cause harm. Tests allow us to look for and find hidden illness, even if the discovery itself may lead patients down a dangerous road. Tests also produce false positive results, sometimes at an astonishingly high rate, leading to unnecessary additional tests, procedures, or treatments that may cause patients substantial harm at an extraordinary cost. But a thorough doctor will look. A thorough doctor will find. And then a thorough doctor will treat. Many studies and books have been written documenting the futility of excessive testing.[169] But a thorough doctor is not discouraged by the negative perceptions portrayed by doubters. If there are medical problems present, despite a patient's age, and despite minimal evidence to support aggressive posturing, we as doctors tend to find those problems and fix them. This is a path that Medicare endorses, as it will pay for tests and procedures more readily than it pays for much else. It is a path endorsed by our society and by so many of my patients. And it is a path that current Medicare reform efforts do little to discourage.

As a doctor, following the route of thorough medicine by ordering a lot of tests is the path of least resistance. Nothing is more difficult than trying to explain and reason through the natural declines inherent to aging, than trying to convince patients and their families in this age of scientific marvel trumpeted by the media and the medical community that a minimalist approach is most sensible, than spending excessive time on the phone or in the office discussing something that can be served to them with far less effort and at a far lower cost for them (if a much higher cost for the system) by writing prescriptions and ordering tests.

The thorough approach to medical care makes people happy, because they think we really care about them. It makes us happy, because we have to spend less time with our patients (since we just write prescriptions for tests and specialist visits and send them on their merry way), and thus can see more patients, giving us more revenue. Lawyers don't sue thorough doctors, families don't yell at thorough doctors, and Medicare rewards thorough doctors by paying them well for their tests and procedures.

No one can deny that the aging process is riddled with incessant decline. For reasons none of us fully comprehend, every part of the body deteriorates simultaneously as people reach advanced age, and even a person who seems to be completely together is really a patchwork of Band-Aids and broken machinery that can be unraveled by one minor insult. I have seen apparently healthy elderly people regress from independent and active members of society into nursing home dependent skeletons in a matter of weeks without any very good scientific explanation as to what exactly precipitated the plunge, and without it slowing despite tens of thousands of dollars of intervention tossed at them. Such a reality frustrates patients and their families. It does not fit well into the neatly packed narrative that American medical lore has painted for them. There needs to be a reason; things don't just happen. Somewhere out there exists a doctor, test, or procedure that can make sense of an older person's decline and fix it. The more we look for problems, the better chance we have of resolving them. Why give up when there is an answer out there waiting for us, if only we keep plugging at it?

## Screening: Prostate Cancer

Mr. L. came to my office for a routine visit. A healthy man in his late eighties, he was independent and vibrant, even if he had slowed down a bit in the last few years. But that did not bother him. He still saw friends and family, took naps when he was tired, did a little reading when his eyes allowed it, and had found a good cocktail of juices and stool softeners to get his bowels moving just about right.

On the day of the visit we both agreed that he had not had a com-plete exam for a while, so we did one, although I must say that none of us physicians really know what a complete exam really is, and there is very little evidence that a "complete exam" is of any validity.[170] But as part of this exam I shoved my lubed finger into his rectum, and there I found a surprise. Mr. L.'s prostate was huge and rock hard.

"Are you peeing OK?" I asked him.

"Sure, every day like clockwork. Sometimes I get up at night, but I go right back to sleep."

I explained to Mr. L. the significance of my finding. Very often large, hard prostates indicate prostate cancer. We could get a PSA blood test to help confirm it, or I could send him directly to a urologist for a biopsy. Or we could do nothing.

"What would you do?' he asked me, hardly concerned about the gravity of what I had just relayed to him.

So I laid out the arguments pro and con. On the one side, even if he had prostate cancer it would likely not kill him at his age, and a bi-opsy was not without its risks. On the other side, if he did have prostate cancer it could be treated, although there was no real evidence that treatment would lead to a longer or better life, and treatment had its own risks. "If you want," I said, picking some nebulous middle road. "We can just get the PSA and see what it is before we make a decision. But it's probably going to be high, and it won't change what we do."

"Then," he said with a smile. "Let's not do anything for now. If I have problems with my pee, I'll let you know." After all, he told me, he was pretty old. I promised him that I would keep my fingers away from his prostate from now on.

A few years passed and Mr. L. meandered down to the office one morning complaining he could not urinate for the past twelve hours. He felt well, but was just concerned. I was rounding in the hospital, and no other doctors could see him in the office, so the front staff made an urgent appointment with a local urologist. It turned out that by the time he arrived there he was able to pass urine; likely he was a bit dehydrated.

But the urologist checked a PSA, as they always do, and the result was an astonishing 150. Now, those of you who understand PSA's know that anything over 4 is high, over 10 is likely cancer, and the highest I had ever seen was about 60. One hundred fifty is beyond conception.

The urologist did some tests and suggested immediate treatment for what he called aggressive prostate cancer, although Mr. L. had no symptoms. He ordered a hormone injection of a medicine called Lupron that curbs the spread of prostate cancer, which Mr. L. agreed to take. Soon after that injection, Mr. L. became profoundly weak. I saw him and could not ascertain a cause. But he deteriorated quickly, and soon we had to put him in the nursing home temporarily to get him stronger.

Mr. L. was almost ninety when that occurred, healthy as can be. He never left the nursing home, and died somewhere close to his hundredth birthday. He also never walked again. He declined further treatment for his prostate cancer, and clearly that cancer did not kill him. Nor did the cancer cause him any harm. Rather the treatment for that cancer did him in. And his story is more common than anyone seems to realize.

Tests are potentially dangerous because they lead to unnecessary treatments that can be toxic. The testing process itself—whether a needle or an x-ray—can cause direct harm to the body and send a frail person into a tailspin. Disease, if left alone, often can coexist with an elderly body. Even cancer may not kill many elderly people; some cancers even regress on their own.[171] A large amount of men die with prostate cancer but not of it.[172] The introduction of PSA screening, followed by invasive testing and aggressive treatments for prostate cancer, has not reduced mortality in the elderly.[173] [174] [175] [176] Many people have breast cancer, skin cancers, even colon cancer and they die of something completely different. Only when we look hard enough and find these cancers do we cause them problems. Unfortunately we do not know who may benefit from screening and who may be harmed by it. We can never know. But as people age, the prospect of finding a problem that can save or improve their lives becomes less realistic, while the prospect of causing injury becomes more common.

I talked earlier in the book about a child who insisted on having PSA measured in her dad. When the PSA was elevated she brought him to a major medical center under the care of experts who continued to test him and measure him, to treat him, and to monitor the treatment. His life became consumed by the screening process, to the point where he physically declined from a deluge of stress. That story evokes two very important points. One is that stress can be a salient result of too much testing.[177] When screening tests reveal problems, then a patient has to live with the reality that some horrible process is ravaging his/her body. That pestering thought is very toxic, and it takes the life out of many of my patients. This is not something easy to measure, but it is a reality I see regularly. The second point is that the testing and treatment process can instigate a substantial decline in quality of life, especially after a prostate cancer diagnosis.[178] [179] [180] A British study showed that most men retrospectively aware of the implications of their prostate screening regret ever getting it.[181]

## When to Screen: The Case of Mammography

In the population at large, finding problems and treating them does not necessarily extend life. Not only do treatments for certain conditions in the elderly such as prostate cancer, breast cancer, pancreatic cancer, lung cancer, etc., not definitively help reduce mortality, but even more revealing is that many people who are treated for these diseases and "cured" tend to die at the same time they would have even if they had not ever been tested and treated.[182]

Many organizations, such as the US Preventative Services Task Force (USPSTF), elucidate the utility of screening tests at certain ages. Mammograms, PSA tests, colonoscopies, etc., are all given age ranges when they are no longer effective in preventing illness. [183] For most screening tests, it has been shown that utility diminishes and harm increases by age seventy-five. Still, despite this reality, Medicare will continue to pay for those tests as well as for the treatment incurred by what the tests reveal, whether the tests are deemed useful or not. CMS has talked about paying only for screening tests approved by the US Preventative Services Task Force, but I doubt that will occur in our current politically charged medical environment, where patient demand for "thorough" care often trumps common sense and when rationing of care has become such a dirty word. The case of mammograms is illustrative of my skepticism.

Several decades ago CMS changed its rules and permitted mammograms only every other year for older women, a decision supported by copious data. But immediately, protests by women's and consumer's groups caused CMS to buckle and revert to the status quo of paying for annual exams at every age. Many researchers question whether the elderly should have mammograms at all. A recent *New England Journal of Medicine* study concluded that most tumors detected by mammograms are not clinically relevant and require no treatment. The study found that 1.3 million women were overdiagnosed in the past thirty years. One thousand women are screened to prevent one breast cancer death, while the screening triggers sixty-three unnecessary biopsies and no proven decrease in overall death.[184] Several other studies similarly cast doubt on mammography as a means of reducing death in the elderly, most notably two by Welch's group at Dartmouth.[185] [186] [187] [188] The most recent study followed 90,000 women for twenty-five years and found no reduction in breast cancer death among women with mammograms compared to those who did not receive mammograms. In addition, because mammograms pick up cancers so early, and since many cancers either grow slowly, do not grow at all, or even regress, the early detection of cancer led to unnecessary surgery, radiation, or even chemotherapy for nonlethal cancers in 2.36/1000 women who received mammograms.[189] A recent op-ed by Welch highlights the uncertainly of screening, pointing to the need for more study to obtain better answers. He cites that among a thousand fifty-year-old American women screened annually for a decade, 3.2-0.3 will avoid a breast cancer death, 490-670 will have at least one false alarm, and 3-14 will have unnecessary treatment. He also notes that many women may not want to be screened if better informed of those numbers.[190] His article was immediately assailed by several physicians, including Barbara Monsees, who chairs the Breast Imaging Commission of the American College of Radiology, and Murray Rebner, President of the Society of Breast Imaging. These authors use relative risk to dramatize the same numbers used by Dr. Welch, stating that "women who get mammograms regularly have a 30 to 45 percent lower risk of dying from breast cancer." They also falsely state that annual mammography is universally endorsed for all women over the age of forty.[191] Clearly, numbers can look dramatic when related as relative risk percentages, but while mammography does save lives, it is at a very low rate and with complications. In our oldest patients, even the prospect of saving lives is very dubious.

No one has demonstrated any significant advantage of screening women over seventy-five years old, who comprise the bulk of my patients. States the USPSTF website: "Among women 75yrs or older, evidence of benefits of mammography is lacking." A 2001 discussion of screening in the elderly suggests that most organizations do recommend that there be an upper age limit to mammography, citing more generally that "Some of the greatest harms of screening occur by detecting cancers that would never have been clinically significant. This becomes more likely as life expectancy decreases."[192] An earlier study finds that the prevalence of detecting clinically significant breast cancer through mammography declines with age, citing the potential harm from finding and treating lesions that will not impact mortality.[193] Some of my older patients ask me what the harm is of getting a mammogram; why not get the test and acquire some information. But there *is* potential for harm. Biopsies are not without risk. Treatments for nonlethal, slow-growing cancers (which are common in the elderly) are very risky. And the many women who are forced to live with the repercussions of false-positive mammograms have heightened levels of anxiety and other untoward psychological trauma. [194] [195] Medicare's quality indicators do not advocate such screening over the age of seventy-five. But Medicare continues to pay for the test regardless of age, and has not used its guidelines to discourage screening mammograms in the oldest patients.

## Screening for Everything

Bone density testing, something that is promoted by clinical guidelines and by Medicare's quality measures for all women over age sixty-five, is a screening test that most of my patients feel is important. But those who get the test, some of them annually, have not considered how they would treat abnormal results, as many refuse to take the medicines that would be necessitated by a diagnosis of osteoporosis. In fact, they are correct to be skeptical of treatment, since Bisphosphonates, the primary means of treating abnormal bone density tests, are of limited efficacy and have many adverse effects,[196] [197] something we discussed in the prior chapter. In addition, no randomized studies have demonstrated long-term benefit from bone density testing.[198] In women with a normal bone density test, it would take fifteen years for 2 percent of them to develop a vertebral fracture,[199] making it questionable to even recommend subsequent testing in such patients. Thus, a well-regarded test that is believed to be a vital part of thorough medical screening, and that is both paid for and *encouraged* by Medicare through its clinical performance measures, does not necessarily lead to any meaningful enhancement of health in the vast majority of people who undergo it, but can expose women to potentially dangerous medicines that could harm them. The test also labels many women with a diagnosis of osteoporosis, so now these women think they have a disease. In fact, by recently changing the definition of what is considered to be an abnormal bone density, more women now think they have osteoporosis, despite the fact that the new definitions of low bone density do not predispose people to additional clinically relevant fractures.[200]

Colonoscopies are also tests that are recommended for many patients but are very controversial in their utility. My grandfather died from a colon prep, so I admit to being a bit jaded. He was in his seventies, had serious heart disease, but still had a colonoscopy for routine screening that showed either a very large polyp or an early cancer, either of which required surgery to remove. So he went to the hospital very healthy, drank the gallon of GoLYTELY solution that night in preparation for the surgery, and was found dead on the floor the next morning. Likely that prep, which tears the body apart by pulling electrolytes from every cell imaginable, pushed his heart beyond his limit. An unnecessary test did him in. Many of my patients have had their bowels punctured by colon screening, being forced to have major surgery and then wear a bag to collect their stool. Some die. I have had other patients discover polyps that may become cancer, and they tout this as lifesaving. But the reality is much different for our elderly,[201] where the risks of serious complications increase dramatically even as the benefits of screening diminish. In fact, it is felt that about a third of all cancer screening in the elderly is inappropriate.[202] [203] These studies and others demonstrate that the number of lives saved from colon cancer detection with colonoscopy (approximately .25/1000 people screened in a year) is lower than the major complications, including perforation, that may result from screening (approximately 2.5/1000 people screened in a year). That is why so many organizations, including the US Preventive Services Task Force, do not endorse colon screening over age seventy-five, something echoed by Medicare's quality indicators. But many patients still believe scopes are necessary, despite their potential harm, and Medicare will gladly pay for the test, any complications that occur because of the test, and whatever treatments may be offered to ameliorate what diseases are uncovered.

The most recent screening test to hit our popular lore is that of CT scans for smokers and ex-smokers flowing from the results of a large randomized study, NLST. I have rarely met a smoker who does not think that he/she may get lung cancer; they often tell me that they would rather die of lung cancer than quite smoking. But now medical science has devised a means of preventing them from having to make that choice. A recent study showed that by performing annual high definition CT scans on smokers and ex-smokers we can detect cancer early and save lives. The truth is much less spectacular[204] when absolute risk reduction is looked at instead of the oft published relative risk reduction, but that did not stop the press from declaring the discovery a triumph of medical science. In fact, despite a 20 percent relative risk reduction touted by the article results, the absolute risk reduction in lung cancer death was eighty-seven people out of 26,722 people screened with three sequential CT scans, although approximately 40 percent of those found to have cancer either had negative CT screens or skipped the screen entirely. This is an absolute risk reduction in lung cancer of 3.3/1000 people screened over five years. Of people screened, almost a quarter had false positive CT screens that were proven not to be cancer after further tests, some of which were invasive and potentially dangerous.[205] The US Preventive Services Task Force, which now recommends CT screening, cites a false positive rate of almost 70 percent, and states that 9/1000 people who are screened are subjected to unnecessary biopsies or surgeries for benign lesions.[206] A subsequent look at the NLST data suggested that 18 percent of all cancers removed were indolent: if left alone, they would have not grown and thus would have caused no harm.[207] Still, the press and many cancer screening organizations now endorse the test, and it is likely that soon enough insurance like Medicare will start paying for CT scans to screen smokers and ex-smokers between 55–79 years old. Time will only tell whether such screening is endorsed by Medicare's quality indicators.

CT screening, then, while showing a small reduction in lung cancer mortality, also confers substantial risk, especially in exposing large numbers of screened people to unnecessary procedures and treatments. It is also unclear if the results obtained in the ideal environment of NLST study centers can be generalized, or if the survival benefit will extend beyond five years, especially since smokers have a higher mortality rate from other causes. But CT screening is of dubious value for other reasons too. For one, the test gives patients the illusion that science is invincible and can cure even the most pestering of problems. Smokers will never expect to die of lung cancer due to the technological brilliance of our medical system, and thus the quit rate may suffer. Secondly, there are multiple risks with scanning. More than half of smokers over fifty years old have nodules on CT scans. Most nodules detected will never become cancers, yet to prove that, patients may undergo biopsies that can pop their lungs, cause infection, and even kill them. There is also no evidence prior to the recent study that following such nodules through serial CT scans is lifesaving or otherwise beneficial.[208] [209] [210] [211] Also, there is a radiation risk associated with CT screening estimated to cause as many as 12/10,000 deaths in smokers screened.[212] Thus, because of an abnormal CT, some patients who do not have disease will be subjected to harm, even death, unnecessarily; many will be labeled with and treated for diseases that are not dangerous; and all are given the false promise that medical science can ameliorate even the most vexing health care issues that plague us. Finally, generalized screening of smokers with CT scans will be very expensive and further tax Medicare while likely providing marginal, if any, absolute risk improvement once long-term data become available.

An editorial by Patrick Hahn in the *Baltimore Sun* states that the cost of "the illusion of cheating death" with lung cancer screening will be in the billions of dollars every year. This for perhaps a marginal extension of life, at best. As Professor Hahn poignantly states about patients who demand such testing: "On the one hand, too many people cannot be bothered to practice the behaviors that don't cost anyone else a penny, and which have proved to promote health and longevity: exercising, eating sensibly, and refraining from smoking and excess drinking. On the other hand, they demand endless, expensive medical interventions—not just regardless of cost, and not just regardless of how great a role their own foolishness has played in bringing on their disease, but regardless of whether said medical interventions are doing anyone any good."[213] To me, that sums it up perfectly. And if Medicare bows to public pressure and starts paying for such testing, even though it does not pay for smoking cessation therapies, then we do not have to look very much past that fact to wonder why it is collapsing.

What little evidence does support screening in the elderly is itself of questionable validity. Screening research tends to recruit better educated people with fewer medical problems, and these studies are subject to multiple biases.[214] One of my colleagues, Erik Rifkin, has written a book about excessive testing. The book, *The Illusion of Certainty*, is must reading for every Medicare recipient. Essentially it explores several diseases, tests, drugs, etc., and, using available data presented in absolute risk/benefit language, determines to what extent testing and/or treatment is beneficial or harmful. It employs the venue of a theater to show how many people will benefit from a specific test or therapy. Dr. Rifkin and I are in the process of writing another book to expand the concept to even more tests and treatments. For instance, the benefit of smokers who quit smoking essentially fills every seat of the theater (they all benefit), while doing a colonoscopy in an asymptomatic person over eighty may fill one seat. But when I show some of my patients the very dramatic theater presentation, they look at the one seat and say, "That one guy could be me. That's why I want the test." I then tell them that there are probably three rows of seats of people who will get serious complications from the colonoscopy, some needing life-long bags to empty their stool due to colon puncture, others dying from the procedure or prep. Still, many patients would rather take that chance. Medicare pays for the test. The doctor recommended it. Their kids insist on it. They don't want to die of colon cancer. And somehow this test, like so many others, will enable them to cheat death. It is a common human flaw to believe such magical thinking. And as long as Medicare is paying, then what the hell.

## X-rays and Other Scans

In our technologically advanced society doctors can employ the power of radiation and magnets (x-rays, CT scans, MRIs, etc.) to look into the body and find trouble. Then, as with numbers that are outside of the "normal" range, we can make everything better again with enough effort, probing, and slicing. Very few see the danger of digging too deep and then repairing what is wrong. Says one doctor who studies health care delivery: "If a procedure or surgery helps you, you proclaim how lucky you are to live in such a medically advantaged country. If it doesn't work or you get hurt, you think your disease is just too much for modern medicine. If you die, your survivors blame the disease, not the procedure."[215]

Mr. L. came to me with back pain. He seemed to have strained his lumbar spine at the gym. He was healthy and vibrant, and we agreed to treat him with some physical therapy and medicines. But the back did not improve, so we ordered a simple back x-ray. Well, the bones were normal, and the back improved, but the x-ray showed some calcium in the abdomen that was in the area of his aorta, and they suggested we order an ultrasound. So we did. And in fact he had a large aneurysm in his aorta. I sent him to a specialist, who suggested that while the aneurysm (called an AAA) had not caused the back pain (which it sometimes can), it was just too big to leave alone. So Mr. .L went for surgery, and Mr. L. died in surgery. A simple back x-ray that should never have been ordered opened Pandora's box. We screen for AAAs, especially in smokers, and we often find them incidentally, but there is minimal evidence that such a proactive approach reduces mortality.[216] As with Mr. L., it is often best to leave well enough alone. That is not to say that all tests lead us down a dangerous road, as in the case of Mr. L. But we should be cautious when we test, because false positive findings and the discovery of diseases that are best left alone can lead to adverse outcomes if pursued. In many of our tests, especially as patients become older, the majority of "positive" results are not helpful, or are frankly harmful.

It is estimated that two-thirds of MRIs ordered contribute nothing to patient care. In fact, like with Mr. L., we uncover "problems" for which we are not searching, leading to more tests, procedures, and potential harm. One study showed that 87 percent of whole body scans found abnormalities, 40 percent required more testing, and less than 1 percent revealed any clinically relevant information after all the testing was complete.[217] In people without any symptoms, random x-rays revealed gallstones in 10 percent of people tested, old strokes in 10 percent, cartilage damage to the knees in 40 percent, and bulging back discs in 50 percent.[218] Knee imaging poorly predicts clinically relevant illness, especially in the elderly, and contributes virtually nothing to help improve outcome or symptoms in patients with knee pain.[219] [220] In addition, despite their limited utility, some studies suggest that the radiation exposure inflicted by such tests as CT scans can actually directly harm patients; the National Cancer Institute estimated that in a single year CT radiation caused 29,000 excess cases of cancer and 14,500 excess deaths.[221] And yet these tests are commonly requested and ordered; they are considered standard of care for many Americans. And Medicare pays for them; I have never seen a request for a scan denied in my twenty years of practice.

Many illnesses, especially cancers, have become more prevalent in our society because imaging and testing have revealed tumors that previously would have been undetected. But although we have diagnosed more cancer, that has not translated to any improvement in survival. For instance, the diagnosis of kidney cancer has increased dramatically from 1975 to the present, but there has been no change in kidney cancer deaths. Some of these increased numbers of kidney cancer were found incidentally on CT scans done for other reasons, and they may not have caused harm, or would have eventually triggered symptoms before leading to problems and more targeted scans. Because so many kidney tumors are identified, many people have had to endure unnecessary, potentially dangerous procedures and surgeries to remove tumors that may have been harmless if left alone.[222] In fact, autopsy studies demonstrate that in 25-40 percent of cases, patients die from causes that differ from their diagnosis,[223] a diagnosis often discovered by a radiologic test that should not have been ordered.

## When to Test: The Case of Back Pain

The perception that MRIs will help a person with back pain is common among my patients, but the data for such a presumption is at best specious.[224] [225] [226] That reality does not stop people from requesting them.

Many of my patients with back pain ask for back MRIs, despite my advice otherwise. There are certainly times when an MRI makes sense: when pain persists despite every effort to curb it, when neurologic damage is evident, and when the test may reveal some finding that is pragmatically treatable. But we should only get the MRI if we are looking for something that can be fixed, and for which the patient is willing to undergo available treatment. Only 1/2500 MRIs provide information that is not uncovered by the patient's history, and less than 1 percent of all scans show cancer, typically in people with either a past history of cancer or who have other symptoms or signs of cancer.[227] Virtually none of these cancers are curable, even if discovered by testing. Overall 75 percent of people with lower back pain make a full recovery within three months without treatment, and there is no change in this number if they have received an MRI.[228] And several studies have demonstrated that there is no improvement in outcome or psychological well-being in people who receive an MRI compared to those who do not; just the opposite may be true. MRIs done within the first month of symptoms can lead to worse outcomes and unnecessary surgery.[229] [230] But why not test and find the precise cause of the pain? After all, it is better to obtain more information and find out what is going on rather than guess. That is thorough medicine.

In fact, when MRIs are done on populations of people with back pain and those without back pain, both groups are found to have similar disc problems in their back regardless of whether they have pain. Ninety percent of **asymptomatic** people over the age of sixty have spinal abnormalities on MRI, including spinal stenosis, bulging discs, and even herniated discs.[231] [232] This is a tremendously high false positive rate. Of course, the patients with back pain claim that the bulging disc uncovered by the MRI is causing their pain, when in fact it may have been there quietly for years and has nothing to do with why they are hurting. If we find a slipped disc, and we have already exhausted common treatments such as physical therapy and medicine, then potentially the patient can have cortisone injections or even surgery. But will that treatment work, and will the patients want that treatment? If the answers are no, then there is no purpose to getting the MRI. Many studies have demonstrated the futility of invasively treating most back pain.[233] [234] One study suggested that 10 percent more people with back pain did better long term without cortisone injections in the back compared to those who had injections.[235] Thus treatment that is performed explicitly as a result of an MRI and which itself carries substantial risk, as we learned from the fungal infected injections that killed people recently, has dubious value and can cause harm, especially since the vast majority of people improve without any testing or treatment. Still, MRIs are ordered routinely, are considered thorough, and are paid for by Medicare without any hesitation.

In the world of medical common sense, certain means exist to evaluate the utility of a test. First of all the test should be performed to look for a specific condition, not to just look around and see what is brewing. When we look around we often uncover conditions not related to the patient's complaint, and that sends us down a very precarious road. Second, the patient should have a high pretest probability of having that condition; in other words, his/her clinical state makes that condition very likely. When the pretest probability is low, then the likelihood is that whatever the test reveals may not be the cause of the patient's problem, or could be false positives. In addition, the test needs to add information that a medical history or physical exam will not reveal. Third, the condition for which we are testing will be harmful if left alone and will worsen without intervention. Fourth, an intervention exists to fix the problem, the patients would want to pursue that intervention, and the intervention is less dangerous than the condition itself if left alone.

Unfortunately, common sense is often absent from both our current dogma of what constitutes thorough medical care and how Medicare finances that care. It is far easier for us as doctors to just order a test than to engage in a complicated conversation with our patients about the ramifications of testing. Medicare will reimburse doctors well for testing, but it does not pay adequately for that type of discussion.

## Cardiac Testing

Cardiac testing is especially illustrative of how Americans perceive tests and procedures as being beneficial despite evidence to the contrary. Many of my patients expect an EKG as part of their annual exam, and many more see cardiologists where they receive regular cardiac testing—EKGs, echocardiograms, stress tests, Holter monitors—as part of routine surveillance. Such testing seems both innocuous and thorough, and most of my patients are glad to be so well cared for by their doctors. However, while 700,000 Medicare patients received treadmill stress tests every year in 2008 (and the numbers continue to climb), such tests poorly predict both who has serious disease and who has no disease.[236] In fact, while 1.9/1000 may have disease detected that if treated will improve their outcome, 6.5 people out of 1000 people with low-risk nuclear stress tests will have cardiac death or heart attack in a year despite being told their tests are normal, and 2/1000 people tested will actually suffer an excessive risk of death, heart attack, and stroke (from unnecessary procedures done based on the very high rate of false positive tests) simply from getting a stress test they did not need. There may even be an increased risk of cancer due to radiation exposure.[237] The numbers are not very different in CT angiograms, which are the newest version of testing people for cardiac disease. Thus, such testing often misses those with real disease, and also causes unnecessary death and disability in people who should never have received the test in the first place.

Mr. S., who is in his seventies, is not a big fan of testing, but he was pushed to have one out of necessity. Not that he was feeling poorly; he was not. He was a pilot who continued to relish trips into the clouds, and he paid for that endeavor by teaching flying lessons at the local airport. He was excellent at what he did, and it gave his life a meaning and purpose that allowed him to thrive. But one day a new FAA doctor looked at his EKG for his annual flight exam and thought it seemed abnormal. In fact, it had always been abnormal, and Mr. S. pulled out a very old EKG to demonstrate that fact. But the doctor insisted on more testing, and he ordered a flurry of tests from a cardiologist, including a thallium stress test, all of which Medicare paid for. Understand, Mr. S. has no heart symptoms, few risk factors, and that the test was done only because of an EKG that had not changed in decades. But when the thallium test was read as being abnormal, now he was told he had a serious illness.

It was not markedly abnormal, and even the cardiologist accepted that it may be a normal variant. So he ordered a CT angiogram, which also demonstrated equivocal results. Then he ordered a cardiac catheterization (itself a potentially dangerous procedure), which showed a blockage of one artery, not necessarily the artery that was suspected to be blocked by the prior tests. Still, the cardiologist recommended surgery to fix the artery, since the narrowing was not amenable to the placement of a stent. Mr. S., knowing that only the surgery would get him in the air again, reluctantly complied.

The surgery proved complicated. Mr. S. has a decades-long platelet problem, meaning that his blood does not clot well. So he bled excessively. Then his prostate expanded and he could not urinate. He needed a urinary catheter placed, and had to go home with it and with nurses to take care of it. When they attempted to remove the catheter, his prostate continued to block his urine flow. This went on for months, until finally he needed another surgery to open the prostate. Over the course of this his stress level escalated, and he became progressively more debilitated. Months passed before he could function well again. And when they checked his heart tests again, there had been no change. Nothing improved. They still denied him his license. The surgery likely did nothing to prevent a heart attack or to extend his life. In fact, it only induced pain and misery, increased his stress and disability, and potentially caused him great harm. A door was yanked open that should have been kept closed. And Mr. S. was the victim of the abuse of thorough.

What is the evidence that cardiac testing—stress tests, echocardiograms, catheterizations—helps reveal problems whose resolution leads to saved lives? When elderly patients are having chest pains or shortness of breath, should they see cardiologists, get procedures, have blocked vessels fixed by stents or surgery? So many of my patients get stress tests on a regular basis, sometimes even every year. Some of them have symptoms, some had symptoms or heart problems in their past, some just want to make sure everything is OK. There are clearly medicines that help prevent heart attacks in patients with certain conditions, some of which may be defined through cardiac testing, so there is a rationale for targeted testing of specific people. We do know that in certain types of heart disease, invasive procedures such as bypass and stenting can be lifesaving.

But the basis for conducting many heart tests may rest on faulty grounds, as we have discussed.[238] Even if one argues that a stress test or echocardiogram can reveal a problem that will lead to beneficial treatment, one still has to follow the rules of what constitutes a reasonable reason for testing, as I outlined above. And that certainly does not justify the frequency of cardiac testing that is being inflicted on many of my older patients. In the elderly, heart disease is omnipresent, but that does not mean it is lethal or even damaging, or that repairing the problem will improve clinical outcome, or even that the procedures used to fix problems are not more dangerous than the problems themselves. Many people have blockages in their arteries, but that does not necessarily mean that they are at risk of cardiac death. Some people, probably like Mr. S., developed collateral circulation around the blockages, and many people who had serious cardiac events such as sudden death had relatively minor blockages (less than 40 percent) not detected by stress testing.[239] But we can find heart disease if we look, even if that heart disease is not clinically relevant and even if the treatment of that disease may cause more harm than good. And we are certainly looking very hard!

Many of my patients have had heart attacks at some time in their lives, from fairly significant events, to minor blockages, to silent myocardial infarctions. In this country, and certainly among my patients, heart attacks lead to intensive hospital stays in specialized cardiac care units where patients are subject to a barrage of tests and interventions.

Many of my patients recount tales of getting to the hospital just in time, being saved by the doctors there, and lauding the thorough care that kept them alive then and for time immemorial. This is a lore that is spun by patients who have been through the technologically advanced cardiac hospital care system, and it is one that they keep with them forever. But is our aggressive posturing after a heart attack as beneficial as my patients surmise? The answer may well be no.[240] After an MI in the United States, doctors perform an increased number of invasive tests and vessel opening procedures (catheters, stents, bypass surgeries) than do doctors in similar patients in Canada, but the one year mortality rate is equal in both countries.[241] The regional variations in this country are also striking. Medicare patients in Texas are 50 percent more likely than those in New York to be catheterized within ninety days of an MI with an added cost of $10,000 per patient. However, despite such thorough care, outcomes are worse in Texas than in New York, with increased death and increased injury. [242] Even in people who have not had heart attacks, doctors in the United States perform excessive numbers of catheterizations, stents, and bypass surgeries for symptoms and conditions for which there is not always medical justification. It is estimated that of the 1.2 million elective cardiac procedures, 160,000 or more are not appropriate. [243]

## Opening Blocked Arteries: Stents and Bypass

If we find a blocked artery, should we fix it in the elderly? Does opening an artery extend one's life, or, like with Mr. S., is it a potentially unnecessary procedure with serious complications that does not extend life or reduce symptoms? So many of my patients are walking around with bypassed arteries and multiple stents. They perceive that they would be dead without those procedures. Much of what we know through the literature would dispute that assumption. In fact, in most situations, inexpensive medicines and lifestyle changes are as or more effective than aggressive and expensive cardiac procedures such as stents and bypass surgery.[244] [245] [246] Some would argue that stents and bypass cause more harm than good, and that looking for and fixing blockages is bad medicine, especially for the elderly. We know too that finding blocked heart valves or leaking valves will not necessarily lead to a treatment that will confer any benefit unless that patient has such severe symptoms that no other option exists. [247] [248] [249] [250] Again, many patients are happy to have such a thorough approach to their care, and Medicare will pay. But the data does not support their optimism. And the result of such excessive testing may be increased stress, medical complications, or even death.

Even when people sail through elective cardiac procedures, and even though they are typically convinced that their lives have been saved by the timely intervention, testing and treatment is not without risk. There is good evidence that people who undergo open heart surgery suffer mental decline.[251] People can bleed, develop cardiac complications, acquire infections, and sustain organ damage from cardiac tests and procedures. Some never regain their prior level of function, especially the old and frail. All patients who undergo cardiac procedures now are labeled as cardiac patients, and this creates a psychological strain that impacts them for the rest of their lives. Some see themselves as being sick, and thus subject themselves to even more tests and procedures, a venture financed by Medicare.

Mr. B. was a good looking, pleasantly demented man in our retirement community who lived from smile to smile and joke to joke. His slick, debonair southern accent (his family hailed from New Orleans where they owned a large part of that city from well before the Civil War) wooed women, young and old, and instigated ire in his wife. He often wandered to the medical center to spend time with us.

Mr. B.'s most pressing medical problem was shortness of breath from a leaky heart valve. He saw a ton of specialists, had an abundance of tests performed regularly, was on a drawer full of medicines (which he took when he felt like it), but nothing fully alleviated his symptoms. He never complained about his breathing; other people were more concerned about it than he was. He took his time getting from one place to another with frequent rests and, as he explained, he had ample time so that was no problem. At the retirement community in which he lived he could do anything he wanted, including frequently visiting us, panting a bit, but always with a smile and a joke. When I asked him if he was OK, he would say, "Sure, I can still play my cornet; when I can't do that, I know I am in trouble."

He always talked about his cornet and the bands he played with in New Orleans. We never knew if he really still played it or whether it was an echo from his past. Then one day he marched down to the medical center with a black box, pulled out his gold trumpet, and belted out some tunes, with a pitch as smooth and suave as Mr. B. himself. Everyone gathered around to listen to his show that he sprinkled with jokes and stories. Mr. B. loved an audience, and he sucked in the attention. On many days after that, he would show up with his cornet.

Although I saw Mr. B. fairly often, typically at the behest of his wife, or as an excuse for him to come down and mingle with the ladies, he never complained. Never. He did not have an ache or pain, never a sad thought, never a flicker of distress. But his wife worried, especially about his breathing. She brought him from specialist to specialist. They pushed her to have him repair his leaky heart valve, something Mr. B. bucked until finally the pressure to be aggressive became overwhelming to him. So he agreed to the procedure, probably just to shut everyone up.

I remember the day before his surgery. Mr. B. walked down to see us with his toothy grin, his smooth one-liners, and his cornet. He played a few tunes for us, never gasping for air, and hung around for a while before meeting his wife at dinner, which started at about 4:00 p.m. That was the last I saw him. Several days later we learned that Mr. B. had died in the hospital. The lifesaving surgery had triggered a cascade of other problems from which he could not recover.

Mr. M. was a short statured man who liked to meander down to our medical center to chat with the receptionists or whoever else was willing to talk. Like Mr. B., he would often toss them a joke or a funny story in his gruff voice. He had been a working man all his life, not particularly well educated or well spoken, but always upbeat and outgoing. His wife, also a bastion of pleasantness, was more reserved, playing the straight man to his comedic routine.

For any number of reasons—small strokes, cerebral atrophy, arthritis, neuropathy, blocked blood vessels in his heart—Mr. M. began to lose his balance and become more short of breath. He fell often, and became unable to traverse long distances, even with a walker. Frequently his wife pushed him to the medical center or to dinner in a wheelchair, something not only demeaning to Mr. M., but also something that threatened his spontaneity and independence. I did the requisite CT scan of his brain and some labs. We ordered physical therapy, played with his medicines, tried some tricks, but his balance continued to decline and his breathing worsened. And so as I often do in such circumstances, I shrugged my shoulders.

"Hey doc, should I see a neurologist or do something else or is this it?" Mr. M. asked me.

I told him the truth. Fifteen years of experience with neurologists taught me a harsh reality: they were excellent at labeling diseases, but terrible at treating them.

"What about my breathing? Could it be my heart, doc? Everyone tells me I should get my heart looked at."

I told him that is was possible. It was also possible that his leg weakness caused him to be unable to exercise, which led him to be out of shape. We could send him to a heart doctor, do some tests, possibly put him on some medicines, but those would have side effects. He may also be sent down a road littered with invasive procedures.

"Then I don't got time for that. You tell me. What do we do?"

Mr. M. eschewed testing and treatments; he was a hands-off kind of guy. Had it not been for the fact that Mr. M. frequently mocked people who rode around the halls recklessly in their electric chairs, then maybe I would have suggested such a chair as a possible solution. I did not. But Mrs. M. did. They bickered about it for several of our subsequent visits, between which Mr. M., determined as ever, tried to walk and nearly broke his hip. Finally, with goading from both of us, he relented. Of course, that was the easy part. I then had to tackle pages upon pages of papers to convince Medicare that an electric wheelchair was justified. That is no simple task. Today it would even be less achievable.

For a while we did not see much of Mr. M. But then one day he emerged in the medical center on his shiny red, brand-new hovercraft wheelchair with which Medicare, after weeks of struggle, had graciously provided him. He mocked himself, pretending to be lame, talking like an old man. And then he showed off his moves, rapid turns, and high-speed sprints down the medical center halls. Soon after that he purchased an electric message display—a smaller version of the screen over Times Square—and welded it to the front of his chair. He became a fixture all over the retirement community. He broadcast holidays, birthdays, events, and even jokes on his chair's display. On various holidays he dressed himself up as Santa, or a leprechaun, or in colonial garb, and he decorated his chair too.

As the years passed, Mrs. M. died suddenly of cancer, and Mr. M.'s health deteriorated. He still pulled himself into that chair every day, always with some purpose like delivering a message or new joke, and he made the rounds, honking his horn to announce his arrival with a smile on his face. The chair allowed him to stay in his apartment and avoid a move to an assisted-living facility or nursing home. Mr. M. died peacefully in his sleep one night. He was in his nineties, and just as happy as the first day I met him.

Medicare paid $5000 for Mr. M.'s wheelchair after a lot of paperwork and arm bending. That wheelchair saved Medicare a ton of cash; one trip to the emergency room for a fall or for shortness of breath often costs much more than that, and a hip fracture or cardiac procedure costs tens of thousands of dollars more. But more importantly, that wheelchair enhanced his life immeasurably and allowed him to preserve his humor and dignity to the end. Had Mr. M. raced from test to test and specialist to specialist, had he been dragged to the emergency room for falls, had he broken his hip and required weeks of inpatient rehabilitation, had he had cardiac tests and stents placed (because certainly if we looked we would have found heart disease that could be treated), Medicare would have paid without batting an eye. Instead Medicare paid for his inexpensive and life sustaining chair reluctantly and after great effort. Contrarily, Medicare paid Mr. B.'s tab without any question or hassle, at a likely cost of tens of thousands of dollars and at the cost of his life.

So often I watch as patients and families make the difficult choices that fell upon Mr. B. and Mr. M. And so often they leap upon the path of thorough care. They try to fix persistent problems, some of which are found by testing and cause no or minimal symptoms, by utilizing the most draconian and invasive methods available. They try to eradicate illness, such as cancers and heart disease, that if left alone are almost always less toxic than the cures. For many patients, families, and doctors the curative, aggressive approach often seems like the right path at first, but rarely does it lead to good outcomes. People justify their decisions by thinking that they have no choice, and indeed the price is often cheaper to the patient to take the most aggressive approach (even if it does cost society a fortune). Medicare makes it easier to be more aggressive; it will not finance help at home and may pay for medical equipment that can improve quality of life, but only after a time-consuming paperwork battle. Contrarily, they will readily pay for tests and procedures, typically with little effort by the patient's doctor. But like with Mr. M., sometimes the least invasive fix is most beneficial. If only Medicare agreed!

## Dialysis

Kidney disease is another illness that is fairly common in the elderly and will be detected if we look hard enough. Many of my older patients have some degree of kidney impairment, and knowing that it will not impact their lives, I typically ignore it. But many doctors are far more aggressive in testing and treating patients with any degree of renal decline. When patients get pushed onto the train of the aggressive kidney surveillance, often at the behest of a kidney doctor (nephrologist) whom they choose to see, they are often barraged by tests, given handfuls of medicines of questionable benefit, and told that dialysis is in their futures. Most of my patients put in this category now have to live with an unnecessary stress that their kidneys can fail at any time. When the kidneys do fail, they are told that they will have to receive dialysis.

Dialysis is not easy, and it is life altering. For three days a week patients go to a dialysis center, have a large needle inserted in a surgically created fistula in their arm, and lie there for many hours as their blood is circulated through an artificial kidney. Very often their blood pressure drops very low, their body chemicals flurry into disarray, and they feel miserable for that day and typically the next. Many of my patients are whisked from the dialysis center to the hospital due to emergencies that dialysis inflicts on their fragile bodies. Some acquire infections or catastrophic difficulties with their shunts. Suffice it to say that while dialysis may be lifesaving for some, it is life destroying for many,[252] [253] [254] and I truly am amazed at how quickly some of my patients are shoved into dialysis with little medical justification for so draconian an approach. Again, as with cardiac patients, many of these patients are thankful for their lives being saved by the miracle of dialysis, whether true or not, and despite the marked decline in life quality many of them must endure, while others truly need dialysis for symptom relief or to stay alive. Still, I have seen demented nursing home residents and weak elderly patients forced to travel to a dialysis center three days a week, wiped out and exhausted, more confused, more ill than before. There seems to be no limit as to who is offered this expensive and debilitating, but very profitable, procedure. And many of them likely would have lived healthy, vibrant lives had they simply been left alone. We have no data to indicate otherwise, and my experience has shown this to be the case.

Medicare pays well for dialysis. In fact, doctors who place their patients on dialysis are likely to be financially rewarded. There are few hard criteria that Medicare requires before dialysis is instigated, and Medicare more readily pays for that procedure than for the much lower cost of helping a kidney failure patient stay off of dialysis machines.

This year I took care of a wonderful man in his eighties who had moved to a local assisted-living facility after starting dialysis. He left friends, including a girlfriend, and a life he truly enjoyed to be closer to his daughter and to a dialysis center. He was emotionally beaten and physically torn apart by the dialysis. I tried to ascertain why he needed dialysis, and why it had to be given three days a week, since that wiped him out almost the entire week. For some reason many kidney doctors insist that anyone who starts dialysis get treatment three days a week, no matter how severe their kidney dysfunction is. I have also found that some people who start dialysis, especially older people, are doing just fine with their poorly functioning kidneys, and it is only excessive testing, excessive medicine use, and specialist involvement that pushes them across the rocky precipice to accept a treatment that is both potentially dangerous and debilitating while often being of questionable clinical efficacy. Mr. B. seemed to fit into that category. He still made urine. His labs were not terrible. He had no fluid overload. Still, his doctors insisted that he needed dialysis and they convinced him and his family that without dialysis his life was in peril. Just a few weeks ago Mr. B. developed problems with his dialysis shunt, the surgically created blood vessel into which a dialysis needle is shoved during treatments. It shut off and became infected, and he needed another catheter placed into his chest to continue his dialysis treatment. He started getting weaker and more depressed. Then, as I learned the other day, he went in for a minor surgery to fix the shunt, and he died.

In reality, Mr. B. was dying before the procedure killed him; his life had been torn apart by his "need" for dialysis. But did he really need it? From my review of his record, he did not. He was put on dialysis because his numbers had become worse, even as he continued to live a happy and vibrant life. If his clinical situation worsened, something that I have found to be relatively uncommon in the very oldest of our patients, he may have chosen to endure dialysis at that junction. Or perhaps he would have preferred a palliative approach with home health aides and fluid management, and he could have remained at home with his friends and his life left intact. Although that less thorough approach is inexpensive compared to dialysis, Medicare is not willing to help pay for it. It was more than willing to pay the total bill for dialysis and for all of Mr. B.'s surgeries, including the one that ultimately killed him. That bill is exorbitant, financially and personally. The cost was the man's happiness, health, and ultimately his life.

## Procedures of all Forms

Like with heart disease and kidney disease, many elderly people have medical problems that are revealed by testing and can be potentially fixed with procedures. Most elderly people urinate too much. Some men have large prostates, some men and woman have spastic bladders. High-tech testing can measure urinary flow and even prostate size. Bladder scopes can examine the inner lining of the bladder, the flow, and the precise squeeze pressures of the various components of the bladder. Patients then can be treated with various surgeries for either the prostate or bladder. Recently a patient of mine received Botox injections in her bladder to help spasm. As a result she had complete loss of urinary function for three months, requiring a permanent catheter. Other patients have bladder lifting surgery, which typically affords them a few months of relief before it collapses again at the cost of exposing their bodies to anesthesia and a surgeon's knife.[255] Typically urinary problems can be diagnosed by doctors like me without any testing, and they can be managed with behavior therapy, minor life adjustments, and the use of pads to soak up leaking urine, and often some generic medicine. When conservative treatment fails, and if the symptoms are sufficiently severe, then we may consider tests and treatments. Medicare pays for the aggressive care without blinking an eye. To get it to pay for diapers is a far more difficult venture!

From painful neuropathy in the feet, to acid reflux and swallowing problems, to arthritis and constipation, we have expensive tests to dig into every issue that is common among the elderly. The tests can help define the problems, label patients with specific diagnoses that they can carry with them in their pockets, and afford these patients confidence that they have been thoroughly worked up for their maladies. Typically the testing doctor will offer patients various treatments, some more invasive than others, and most only questionably effective. Many elderly people in our society live with an assumption that if a disease can be defined, then it can be ameliorated. But such thinking is financially costly and medically risky. Prunes help constipation, and exercise certainly helps arthritis; we do not need sophisticated tests and scientific explanations to figure that out. Unfortunately in our test crazed society, common sense and an acceptance of aging quickly evaporate when more technologically sophisticated methods are so readily available for free.

There are of course many examples where testing and treatment make sense and produce favorable results. I have seen people undergo bypass surgery due to persistent pain and shortness of breath that cannot be relieved with medication and behavior changes, and the result is an improvement in their quality of life. One patient who did everything to avoid cardiac surgery, including taking far too many medicines and driving an electric cart, simply had a disease far too severe for him to flourish, preventing him from sleeping at night, going to the bathroom, and visiting his wife at a nursing home. When finally he made the decision to have surgery, he did so because he preferred death over his current condition. The surgery allowed him to function again, and although he only lived another year before he died, he told me that it was the best year he ever had. The price tag for that surgery was high, and it did not buy him extra time to live, but it at least did accomplish something positive.

Similarly, I have had patients who get dizzy and pass out with high frequency, and after testing they are often found to need pacemakers. Those pacemakers can essentially cure them. One of my patients walked around with a heart rate in the 40's and felt tired. For years he fought getting a pacemaker, but when he finally ended up in the hospital due to passing out, and he agreed to have the pacemaker placed, he woke up with more energy than he had had since he was a kid. Another patient fainted incessantly, and thousands of dollars of testing and even a few hospital visits did not define what caused her to do so. Finally, after she passed out while driving and hit a tree, breaking several bones, a monitor in the emergency room happened to show that her heart periodically stopped for several seconds. She had a pacemaker placed, and never passed out again.

Other patients become dysfunctional from arthritis, and despite multiple conservative treatments are unable to live with any quality. For many, joint replacements give them the ability to live again. Some patients need procedures to dilate their esophagus periodically to help them to swallow, and only with testing and treatment can that be achieved. Many patients develop a condition where they stop breathing at night (sleep apnea), the results of which are fatigue and heart strain. Testing and treatment (wearing a very difficult to use mask at night called a CPAP) can help dramatically. Sleep apnea is a good example of how testing and treatment can help, but also how it is bereft of nuance. Very often patients can cure their sleep apnea by losing weight, and no test can help with that. Certain behavior therapies can help too. And very often, despite all the testing they have to endure, my patients refuse treatment, because the treatment itself can be very uncomfortable. And that brings us to where we started. We have to accept that certain maladies are common with age. Many of them can be mitigated and improved by accommodating them and carrying out simple behavioral changes. When they become too much of a burden, and when testing is done for a specific reason that may lead to a treatment that the patient is willing to accept and that is medically beneficial and safe, then that testing makes sense. But tests should not be done simply to be thorough. The pursuit of thorough is a prevalent, dangerous, and expensive idea that has no place in our geriatric medical dogma, even if Medicare is willing to pay.

## Fishing: The Case of Dementia

Sometimes with age the body declines not only organ by organ, but also more globally. My oldest patients are more tired and more confused, they lose weight, they have less desire to interact and get out of their chairs, and they have a litany of complaints for which a cause cannot be ascertained. Often those problems emanate from their medical ailments or their medicines; people with poorly functioning hearts, for example, can experience fatigue and confusion from both the heart and the drugs. Also quite frequently those problems are a manifestation of depression, which itself can be very difficult to treat although always worth a try. But many patients and families demand a more precise and thorough investigation into the physical and mental decline that occurs so frequently in the aged. Somehow, they reason, these symptoms are treatable, and something is underlying them. They want more answers.

"I want dad to have a whole body CT scan to figure out what is going on."

That retort, which is common in many renditions, is a request for us to go fishing. Let's throw our hook into the bay and see what we can snag. Then let's fix whatever we snag, and see if that resolves the problem. If dad does not improve, we will keep throwing in our hooks, maybe even moving to different bodies of water, finding different captains to help us, never backing down until dad gets better, like he was in the past. There is a solution if we are persistent and thorough enough.

Of course, disease specific testing is itself problematic and must be done with care and common sense, but fishing is a geriatric nightmare. It seems to be most common among my most frail and demented patients, typically those whose families have taken over their care, and it causes my patients stress and anguish rather than leading to any meaningful improvement.

Dementia is a prime example of how fishing is used to snag an imaginary resolution to a horrible ailment. When people become confused they may have simple memory loss common in aging, or they may have a progressive form of memory loss called dementia. Medical scientists have defined various forms of dementia, from Alzheimer's disease, to multi-infarct dementia (multiple tiny strokes), to Lewy body dementia (dementia with Parkinson's features), to frontal lobe dementia (striking mostly the front part of the brain and causing more behavior issues). As a geriatric doctor I find these categorizations to be unhelpful. First of all, there is no way to differentiate one from another based on hard evidence. Secondly, I have very few patients who fit into only one category, making me believe that dementia is more of a spectrum of disease that is most impacted by where it hits the brain the hardest. And thirdly, whatever minimal treatments exist for these conditions are virtually the same regardless of how dementia is labeled.

Still, patients and families seeking to better understand the cause and nature of the disease, to better be able to grapple with its progression and to better be able to treat it, want concrete and scientific answers. Some of my patients' families run mom to neurologists, often seek "experts" in academic medical centers, put mom through a battery of tests, and then come to me and announce that mom does not have dementia like I had told them, but rather she has Pick's disease (a form of dementia). I then ask how it is being treated. They proclaim that the experts are putting mom on medicines that will help slow the disease, and that they intend to monitor mom closely. Of course I have to just nod and smile, since I know there is no meaningful way to monitor mom, that the medicines that she is being put on are identical to ones that had previously been ineffective, and that more likely than not the medicines will not impact the disease meaningfully, as I have discussed in the prior chapter.

Just yesterday I was listening to a new NPR show when the host announced that in the next segment we would learn why if you or your loved one has been diagnosed with Alzheimer's disease you may want to get a second opinion. The host then interviewed an academic neurosurgeon who quite bluntly stated that 5–10 percent of alleged cases of dementia are misdiagnosed and are actually cases of NPH (normal pressure hydrocephalus), a condition of fluid build-up in the brain that is treated with a surgical procedure carried out by specialists such as the doctor being interviewed. The doctor explained that with treatment his patients shed their dementia and weakness and became normal again, sometimes instantly.[256]

In my twenty-year experience, I am aware of approximately five patients diagnosed with NPH among the thousands of dementia patients I have cared for, and none of them improved with treatment. Talking to other geriatric doctors, we all have similar experiences. In fact, thorough testing, such as that performed by dementia specialists, will uncover a reversible problem in 3/1000 people with dementia.[257] Much if not all of that testing has already been ordered by primary care doctors like me. We typically perform scans to look for NPH, and we order lab tests to find other possible reversible forms of dementia. Then, when those tests reveal nothing of substance, we have to confront the realities of dementia. Stories like this on NPR only send patients and their families on a quest for the impossible, one that typically ends in disappointment, if it ends at all. As we try to help our patients and families cope with dementia, the press, friends, and a few overly sanguine doctors tell them that they may not have dementia at all. Just find another doctor and miracles will occur!

Dementia is a terrible ailment. Certainly there must be tests for it. There must be treatments. We in this era of scientific advancement cannot sit idly by as mom's brain starts to decay. And as a doctor, if I do not buy into that line of thinking, I am looked at as either someone who is ignorant or as someone who is just giving up; families have accused me of being both many times. But in fact when testing will not accomplish something meaningful, and when no reasonable treatment exists as a result of that testing, I believe that being "thorough" leads us down a dangerous road. Families and patients are flooded with false hope. Many of them believe that they are making progress and that testing did make a difference. Especially with dementia medicines, the placebo improvement rate is very high, as we have discussed. But patients are stressed by the process, something I have seen over and over in my practice, and that stress only exacerbates their dementia and detracts from their quality of life. Fishing for answers is not a very useful means of spending taxpayer funds, although many think is defines thorough, and although it is consistently paid for.

Excessive testing is rewarded in many ways. Financially it is a boon to the doctors who perform the tests. Doctors who place stents into blocked arteries, put people on dialysis, and who cure NPH all are paid very well for their efforts. I once worked with a gastroenterologist who performed 10+ colonoscopies every morning, in many of which he did not visualize the entire colon for logistical reasons such as a poor colon prep. His patients called him very thorough, and he was paid quite well for those tests. Most gastroenterologists I have known are far more scrupulous, but they are still paid more to perform a test than to say no. And patients often prefer a thorough doctor who will say yes.

Much of the push for testing emanates from my patients and their families, not from specialists or doctors interested in making another buck. Medicare enables patients to be tested as often as they wish, by as many doctors and "experts" that they choose to see. Regardless of the need, Medicare will pay as long as we can provide a diagnosis, and that is often the easiest road for doctors and patients to take. It is also seemingly the most thorough. Especially with my frail and demented patients I frequently will offer less thorough advice, such as to increase exercise, eat more protein and fruits, and get out of the apartment and socialize with people. But these solutions reek of surrender. Medicare will not pay for my patient to join a gym and have a personal trainer and nutrition counseling, and it will not finance day care for those who are demented so they can be more active and social. It will also not finance palliative care if they are not near death. This may include home health support, various types of medical equipment, and alternatives to hospitalization, all of which are relatively inexpensive and medically effective while achieving high patient satisfaction. But it will pay for tests and procedures, and it will pay for a patient and family's unending quest to delve into aging's many unfortunate manifestations of decline, despite the high cost and limited utility of such a thorough approach.

Tests and procedures, when not wisely ordered, are dangerous because they help perpetuate the illusion that we can reverse aging by looking hard enough. Not only is such magical thinking endemic in our society, but it is one fully endorsed by Medicare itself. Medicare rewards doctors who test, and it rewards patients who undergo tests, because tests lead to diagnoses, and everything Medicare ultimately pays for is diagnosis driven. Tests often are necessary, if conducted under the umbrella of common sense and reason. But very often in the elderly they are not helpful and are potentially harmful, yet that does not curb their excessive use.

While Medicare seeks solutions to save itself from financial collapse by forcing doctors to squander time and effort adhering to quality care protocols that are of unproven value, it does not place the same standards on its own willingness to pay for tests and procedures that are frequently needless or even harmful. The fact, as we have discussed, that 25 percent of Medicare's total budget is squandered in the last weeks of someone's life, paying for tests and procedures in the hope of reversing the ravages of age without there being any meaningful hope of recovery, is a testament to the futility of Medicare's priorities and payment model. It is also a manifestation of the increasingly specialized medical society in which Medicare now exists, as we will explore in the next chapter.

# 3

# EXCESSIVE SPECIALIZATION, EXPECTATION, AND LITIGATION

*"What's absolutely certain is that we don't need more*
*specialists, but we do need more generalists."*
Shannon Brownlee, *Overtreatment*

With the explosion of medicines, tests, and procedures that can probe and promise to repair every bothersome symptom or clinical abnormality that may riddle an elderly body has emerged the concept of specialization. At the dawn of Medicare most elderly patients were cared for by their trusted primary care doctors, rarely needing to see any other health care practitioners. But now that scenario has reversed. America trains and retains more specialist doctors than primary care doctors, and patients see specialists with increasing frequency. Older patients often are being treated as a series of conditions and diseases, each one confronted independently of the whole person, and each one deserving of the most rigorous attention.

Specialization is a concept based on two essential assumptions. First is the idea that it is best to treat each medical problem independently and aggressively to achieve maximal outcome, typically by an expert in that domain. Such thinking promotes the notion that by fixing numbers, determining precise scientific causes of ailments, and then repairing all that is wrong, our patients will be healthier. Viewing every ailment and condition under a myopic lens allows the doctor to concentrate on that problem and to better manage it. This is compartmentalization of care. Under such a model, we can tackle problems without regard to how they may impact other conditions in the body, because our focus is only on that one condition. For instance, we can assault blood pressure without concerning ourselves with how our treatment may influence falls, fatigue, kidney function, bladder incontinence, and quality of life; those are not within the purview of the blood pressure number and can be handled at another time or by another doctor. We can order multiple tests to determine the cause and effects of high blood pressure, refer to specialized doctors for each problem we may uncover, utilize various drugs and other treatments to drive down the blood pressure and ameliorate its consequences, and concentrate the entirety of our energy on the singular purpose upon which we are focused. Such a model can be utilized to manage other symptoms and conditions such as diabetes, memory loss, fatigue, poor balance, incontinence, and heart disease, each one attacked independently from everything else.

The second assumption flows from the first. With specialized care, we do not have to accept the inevitability of aging, but rather with a directed purpose can reveal what is causing the many symptoms and conditions that emerge as people age and then effectively treat them. In other words, specialization assumes that if we ask why each problem is occurring and point our efforts to resolving the cause of the problem, then we can fix the problem and improve outcome. Memory loss, for example, is not a foregone conclusion with aging. There are a plethora of tests that can be conducted, experts to be consulted, drugs and treatments to try. Typically we can even define the cause of the memory loss more precisely and scientifically. Dementia is too vague a term; with enough testing and probing we can ascertain the precise form of dementia, and possibly even discover some root causes and novel treatments. When one approach to treatment fails, there is likely another doctor, another test, another drug that may nudge us in a more promising direction.

Specialization raises our expectations and encourages us to never give up, because somewhere out there is a reason and resolution if we just push hard enough.

Specialization, then, runs counter to the idea of palliative care, which we have discussed. In a palliative model, especially when directed toward our oldest patients, we only ask questions and probe for answers if the resolution can provide a high likelihood of improved outcome for the patient as a whole. For instance, with memory loss, we may do a few basic tests that can elucidate easily treatable causes of dementia, and even try some medicines for a brief period if they produce clinically meaningful improvement and lack side effects, but short of that we will accept the memory loss, not feel obligated to further label it if such precise definitions do not facilitate better treatments, and then work with patient and family to manage it. With hypertension we will treat blood pressure only until the medicines instigate significant side effects, or until they interfere with other problems or symptoms exhibited by our patient, perhaps being more aggressive if the elevated pressure is imparting a clinically important risk to our patient, such as a stroke risk in someone who has had several strokes or a risk of hemorrhage in the eye. We are not concerned with sporadic elevations in blood pressure, since that scenario has a small absolute risk of impacting our patient's life, while the treatment may have adverse effects. There is an underlying assumption in palliation that aggressive testing and treatment of chronic conditions and numbers will likely not impact the overall outcome of survival in the majority of our elderly patients, and should be primarily done to help our patients feel and function better. That is the very antithesis of a specialized model.

Medicare encourages specialization in several ways. Most fundamentally, it pays for specialized treatment without any pause. If you want to see ten specialists and travel from one medical center to another, there is no limitation imposed by Medicare; all of it will be paid, no referral or permission needed. If your new neurologist wants another brain MRI, even though your primary care doctor ordered one a week ago, then Medicare will pay, no questions asked. And if then you travel to a medical center where another team of doctors wants to repeat the test again, as well as several others, regardless of whether those tests or consultations have any likelihood of impacting treatment, then those too will be paid for. Contrarily, Medicare is much less willing to pay for palliation. While obtaining an few MRIs, an annual carotid ultrasound, an EEG, several pages of blood tests, three consults, and some medication trials is all smiled upon by Medicare, at a cost to the taxpayer of many thousands of dollars and with the potential peril of causing side effects and unnecessary interventions, treating the dementia with physical exercise in a gym, brain programs such as luminosity, a few days a week in a day-care center, and even some home health aides to provide companionship and to help alleviate care giver stress are not paid for at all by Medicare. We can search and test interminably under Medicare's umbrella, with cost and outcome being inconsequential, but we cannot manage the problem, even if such management is both effective and economical. In fact, partially due to the changes from the Affordable Care Act, even the act of helping patients to get a simple wheelchair requires an act of God, pages of papers, and criteria often impossible to satisfy, yet that wheelchair may allow a demented person to get out of the house, to be less agitated, and to avoid expensive and debilitating hospitalization at a tiny cost.

Medicare also encourages specialization by promoting the dramatic explosion of specialty care within our medical landscape. As we will discuss, specialists get paid far more than primary care doctors under Medicare's reimbursement system, and those who perform procedures are remunerated even more generously, thus incentivizing a model of procedure oriented specialization that has become common in the geriatric universe and that is very costly to the system without producing improved outcomes. Because of the financial gap between primary care and specialty care in this country, we have a significant shortage of generalist doctors and an abundance of specialists. By rewarding specialization financially, Medicare has helped it to become the norm in geriatric care. As we will show, the assumptions underlying specialization are often erroneous, and thus the bloated model of care that has emerged under Medicare's auspices has falsely raised expectations while actually impeding efficacious care of the elderly, a formula that has directly contributed to Medicare's financial woes.

My grandmother, who had virtually no serious medical problems, saw multiple specialists and no primary care doctor. Medicare allowed unfettered access to specialty care, even though she enjoyed good health. She urinated too much, so she saw a urologist. She had pain, so she saw an orthopedist and a rheumatologist. She had the shakes, so she saw a neurologist. She could not see and hear well, so she saw an ophthalmologist and otolaryngologist. She continued seeing my grandfather's cardiologist even though she had no heart problems. And I think she saw a gastroenterologist for a little icing on the cake. What struck me as a doctor in training was watching her march to her squadron of specialists with such regularity that those visits became a large part of her life. And when I asked her why she did not have a primary care doctor, my ninety-year-old grandmother bluntly told me that it would be senseless to see one doctor who knew a little about everything when she could see experts in every field.

The visits did not come without a price. Forget the thousands of dollars Medicare paid for her unnecessary foray into the world of thorough medicine, and the fact she had to financially contribute nothing at all. More significantly, she was given inappropriate medicines on several occasions that directly led to harm and to hospitalization, and she was exposed to potentially dangerous tests and to drug interactions. Her neurologist thought she might have Parkinson's (which even as a medical student I knew she did not have), and he started her on a medicine to cure it, a medicine that made her hallucinate. She called my father one night and told him that there were birds in her room having a party. Off she went to the hospital. Several months later her urologist gave her the same medicine, with the same results, landing her back in the hospital. In the end, her death was triggered by a medicine that she should have never received, given to her by a specialist who was concerned about helping the pain in her back but who was not wise enough to know how his treatment would impact the rest of her body. And in the end, too, she spent the last few days of her life in the intensive care unit of a hospital at a cost of thousands of dollars a day, and were it not for the strength and wisdom of her son—my father—she could well have been there far longer with an outcome that in no way would have been good.

## Specialists

Specialists are part of the reason that the American medical system is one of the best in the world when it comes to complex and serious medical problems. America boasts some of the best trained and capable specialists of every discipline, and I am always thankful that there is a willing specialist available when I need one for my patients. In my experience most specialists are superb doctors who happen to be trained to master a small set of problems. Someone who is very ill, or has a medical problem requiring a procedure or a specific expertise, often does need specialty care.

The problem with specialization in the elderly is not related to very ill patients who need intense procedure oriented care. Rather, it occurs when patients have fairly simple and straightforward problems, such as diabetes or hypertension or stable heart disease, problems that can be easily managed by a primary care physician. In our society, with so many specialists and so few primary care doctors, patients with simple chronic issues often see specialists frequently, leading often to redundant care and to very narrowly focused care for each individual problem. Sometimes such care is prompted by patients themselves, who want experts for each of their ailments, sometimes by very busy primary care doctors who look to get some help in managing some of their elderly patient's litany of problems. All of this is paid for by Medicare.

In my opinion, and the opinion of other doctors, the most salient purpose of specialty care is to have experts treat people with complex problems, not to follow uncomplicated chronic ailments. Consequently, I have seen many specialists refer simple problems back to their primary care doctors, while turning away older patients who request colonoscopies, stress tests, and chemotherapy. Contrarily, I have seen many generalists buy into the specialized model of care, referring patients to specialists for every one of their ailments, and even tossing medicines and tests at older patients every time one of them complains about a symptom or exhibits an errant number. Specialization is a mind-set, a manifestation of the concept of thorough, a need to fix numbers and nuisances one organ at a time without having to contend with the broader ramifications that treatment triggers. Most specialists I know would prefer to see more complicated patients rather than the deluge of routine visits that our specialized society tosses in their laps.

When people are young and healthy they develop more unusual and severe diseases that require intensive management by specialists. In fact, young people who do get sick rarely have to see primary care physicians. But when they are older, and every organ begins to deteriorate simultaneously, when function and memory declines, and when quality of life is more impacted by medical intervention than is duration of life, then a more palliative and holistic approach makes sense for the management of chronic medical problems. Specialization of care removes one problem from the rest of the body. So while specialized doctors may insist that LDL cholesterol be kept below 70 as some clinical guidelines suggest (or under 100 as Medicare's quality indicators cite as good care), pounding their patients with statins, and insist that Coumadin levels in patients with A-fib remain strictly within the parameters elucidated by clinical guidelines, ordering frequent lab checks and dose changes to prevent a stroke, and push patients' blood sugars down with more and more medicines, having patients check their finger stick sugars incessantly, they need not be concerned about the patient's lethargy and incontinence and osteoporosis and leg weakness and depression and dizziness and memory loss and stress, some of which are made worse by the treatments they prescribe. They can concentrate all their efforts on a problem or two and "fix" those problems intensely, even if their patients become weaker and more confused as a result.

As a generalist my view must be broader. I cannot worry about whether a patient's LDL cholesterol falls into some preordained range, because when juxtaposed against all his other problems and concerns I know that such fine tuning will achieve no useful clinical outcome, may limit my ability to treat bigger problems that impact the patient, and can often cause side effects that impair quality of life and function. I also know that if I grapple with every minor numerical deviation and problem, despite what the clinical guidelines or a few narrow studies of relative risk suggest, I will flood my patient with medicines, test him excessively, and shift the patient's focus away from what may be more important. So for my patient with high LDL, even though he may have had a heart attack ten years ago and the data demands that he needs to be on a statin (with its impressive relative risk reduction but negligible absolute risk reduction), I may suggest he get off his cholesterol medicine if he has leg weakness and confusion (possible side effects of the drugs), advising him that we no longer check his cholesterol or worry about it.

My goal as a generalist is to prioritize problems and not focus on number fixing and on marginal interventions that will not help my patients remain happy, active, and independent and that may augment side effects. When my patients have fourteen problems, and come to me on twenty medicines, I can more globally see how fixing one problem impairs another, and how so many pills with so many interactions and untoward side effects do not move my patient toward any beneficial outcome despite an improvement in the numbers. After discussing it with patients or their families, I am often able to keep my patients away from tests and procedures that may open up more cans of worms and reveal problems that are dormant in their bodies and are best left alone. I try to focus more attention on how they are doing now and how they can improve their health through exercise, diet, and socialization. For older patients, trying to extend life and erase problems through thorough intensive medical care is not a goal that often can be realistically achieved, and when confronted with everything at once, we generalists can grasp that reality and work with it. While we are not nihilists when it comes to medical intervention, we are very careful to assure that what we do has purpose.

Unfortunately what we generalists often inherit are patients bouncing from doctor to doctor, on a multitude of medicines and undergoing copious procedures, with no one doctor able to treat the patients as a whole or to convince them that backing off may help them feel better.

## The Ramifications of Specialization

Specialized care can have adverse consequences for our elderly. The bloated specialist supply in our country may actually be impairing the health of our elderly, often because there are just not enough primary care doctors.[258] In areas with fewer primary care doctors compared to specialists, older people fare worse in their treatment of cancer, stroke, coronary artery disease, and overall death rate.[259] Overall in parts of the country with an overabundance of specialization, there is a substantial increase in cost of care, hospitalization, and doctor visits without any significant improvement in outcome.[260] Using Medicare data, Fischer and Wenberg from Dartmouth show that in highly specialized areas of the country older people are less healthy and they die earlier despite similar risk factors. They estimate that 30,000 elderly Americans die each year due to excessive care.[261] Also, regions with more specialists report more medical errors, especially in the hospital.[262 263] Again, this is not the fault of specialists, but rather of specialization.

Specialization can medicalize aging, creating an impression that certain conditions that are common in the elderly can be either stabilized or eradicated with focused care that may include aggressive testing and treatment as well as more medicines to manage abnormal numbers and ailments. Specialization draws patients and families into an arena of exaggerated expectations and convinces them that without focused care their medical condition may be far worse. As they age, and as their own capacities for self-decision and function declines, their dependency on specialization does not wane; families often latch onto specialization in their quest to cure their loved ones' declines, sometimes with deleterious consequences.

Mrs. W. had dementia. We ascertained that fact, put her through some basic tests, and even tried a dementia medicine that I stopped due to side effects. Mrs. W.'s daughter wanted to be aggressive in assaulting the dementia and not let it fester and progress. She had read a lot on the Internet about treatments that could slow or reverse the flow of the disease, and she could not understand why I was being so lackadaisical in treating her mother's horrible memory loss. I suggested a more holistic approach: more social interaction perhaps through a day-care program, more exercise, and the implementation of strategies to help curb untoward behavioral outbursts. But Mrs. W.'s daughter felt that that was giving up. Mrs. W. saw a neurologist, who ordered more extensive tests, repeating some I had already done, and put her on more drugs. Now the dementia was labeled as frontal lobe dementia, something her daughter felt obligated to explain to me, as if I had been unable to arrive at her mom's true diagnosis. She regularly brought her mother to the neurologist, who by the daughter's own account was a leader in his field, a dementia expert, and a professor at a major academic institution. She also brought her mother to various other specialists regularly. She continued to see me and give me the reports from those more skilled physicians. Her mom was now on a large amount of medicines. She became sick frequently, possibly from the medicines, possibly from stress, possibly from other conditions that consumed her aging body. These illnesses often drove mom to the hospital, where more tests were conducted to solve each problem that popped up one after another, leading to trips to more specialists and to more tests and more medicines. When her mom's mental decline accentuated, the daughter became disenchanted with her formerly brilliant neurologist and dragged her to yet another neurologist, and started dabbling into alternative medicines and herbal pills about which she became an expert from studying the Internet and taped episodes of Dr. Oz. Eventually Mrs. W. faded from my practice; I think her daughter found another primary care physician, or perhaps none at all, or maybe had to place her in a nursing home. The search for a cure through specialization did not help Mrs. W.; in fact, to me, it hampered a more reasonable approach to dementia that may have provided Mrs. W. and her daughter a higher quality of life.

The search for a dementia cure is irresistible for many patients and families. We have discussed already the futility of finding a reversible cause of dementia even with extensive testing, and we talked about the very modest impact that dementia drugs have on those who suffer from dementia, often producing no significant clinically significant functional improvement, which persists only for a few months in a minority of patients, and that can be associated with serious side effects. Still, I have seen specialists order an abundance of tests, prescribe drugs at high doses and in multiple combinations, and promise that their approach is thorough and effective. More recently Brain Attack centers have littered the medical landscape, where, after extensive high priced testing, various tools and treatments, paid in full by Medicare, are alleged to prevent and reverse dementia. Some such centers use unproven high tech treatments at frequent intervals, prescribe unproven drugs and supplements, and label patients with clinically suspect diseases, all as they purport to be aggressively assaulting a disease that at present has no cure. Hope often trumps reality as so many of my patients and families pursue a specialized aggressive course that leads nowhere beyond frustration, a course that Medicare finances, that the press applauds, and that the public believes to be thorough and miraculous.

Mrs. A. was in her nineties and loved her many specialists, especially her heart doctor, who was a devoted and personable physician. I never could ascertain why she started seeing him in the first place; she had no cardiac history and disdained medicines. Mrs. A. lived with a high blood pressure for over a decade, if not more; numbers of 230/110 were not uncommon. She felt well and was clearly healthy, going to the gym every morning and socializing with friends most of the day, so I never chased those numbers. But her specialists were uneasy, and incessantly put her on blood pressure medicines, fearing she would otherwise get a stroke. Soon after that, she started fainting and feeling tired. She even went to the hospital on numerous occasions after fainting, where she received more tests and more medicines. She saw a neurologist, who looked for other causes of the dizziness through tests and labs. Somehow, even after she and I talked and we agreed to eliminate her blood pressure medicines, she always landed back on them. She, like many of my patients who see specialists regularly, had annual tests, such as heart tests and blood tests, some of whose results were abnormal, which prompted more testing and treatment. The tests and their results made her nervous, but she continued to pursue whatever her doctors asked of her. And she continued to faint every time she went back on her pressure medicines.

I had another patient recently who was an elderly diabetic on insulin. She felt tired and had several episodes of low blood sugar, causing her to be miserably ill. She checked her sugars frequently, being almost obsessed with the fluctuation of her numbers. I felt her sugars were too low, but her diabetes doctor felt they were too high and continued to prompt her to eat better and take more insulin. Finally I convinced her to try less insulin, and then no insulin, and even to check her sugars less. She felt terribly guilty for doing it, afraid she was letting her diabetic doctor and herself down, and that she might get very ill from her misbehavior, even losing a leg or having a stroke. But she felt better, and her A1C sugar level remained decent, although much higher than her diabetic doctor wanted. She never did tell her sugar doctor about it; it was our little secret.

Another of my patients had worsening kidney function by labs, but had no specific abnormalities to indicate he needed dialysis, and was actually feeling quite well. In fact, his labs had been very stable over many years. Still, he was convinced that his kidney doctor believed that he was on the verge of dialysis and that any deviation from the doctor's meticulously detailed instructions could cause instant doom to his sickly kidneys. My patient would not even eat a banana or grapefruit, although he very much wanted to. He watched every morsel that entered his mouth, swallowed a handful of minerals and medicines, and, as per instructions of his kidney doctor, made frequent trips to his cardiologist and endocrinologist to assure that his blood pressure and sugar were also tightly controlled lest they precipitate his cascade toward dialysis, even if doing so made him feel even worse. Nothing I could say convinced my patient that such intensive management was not in fact helping him, when so many others told him that it was. He became consumed by a set of illnesses that were more phantom than real in any meaningful medical context, and his foray into the world of medical specialization certainly detracted from his quality of life without necessarily helping him to be healthier. Still another of my patients had a dialysis shunt put in his arm a year prior because his kidney doctor convinced his wife that dialysis was imminent. The man was severely demented and exhibited many concerning declines in his function, but his wife now had to worry and fret about dialysis and kidney failure, even though his kidney numbers, although abnormal, had not changed in years. She certainly did not need that extra stress, and it was very unlikely that any kidney intervention would improve either the quality or duration of her husband's life.

Specialization can be lifesaving for acute illness, as we have discussed. But there is very little reason for specialists to follow patients regularly for stable conditions, especially as they age and have so many concomitant medical problems, when the treatment of one issue can worsen something else. Still, many patients appreciate such care, Medicare pays for it without question or the need of a referral, and with an abundance of specialists in our society, coupled with the higher revenue that procedure based medicine generates, it is no wonder that specialization has become the norm for older patients with chronic illness.

## The Cost of Specialization

Lower back pain is a prime example of how specialization impacts cost of care. We have discussed the large numbers of unnecessary MRIs ordered for lower back pain, an expense that does not improve outcome.

Many patients also prefer to see lower back pain "experts" such as chiropractors and orthopedic surgeons. Evidence suggests that people who pursue specialized care for their back pain do not fare any better than people who see their primary care doctor, but that the cost escalates substantially.[264] In my experience, back pain experts order more tests and lucrative procedures (such as epidural injections) rather than focusing on more common sense approaches (weight loss, exercise, lifestyle changes) that may ultimately remedy the pain. Of course, patients do not travel to see back pain experts to be told to lose weight; they want the MRI and epidural injection. So we certainly cannot blame the specialist.

That specialists are paid more for each visit and procedure by Medicare than are primary care doctors is an inequity derived by the specialist-dominated American Medical Association Board that recommends payment to CMS, as we will discuss. But some specialists also generate funds indirectly due to the procedure oriented nature of their work. A recent *New York Times* article looked at the cost of colonoscopy, a procedure that increased in frequency by 50 percent between 2003 and 2009. Although Medicare's direct payment to the specialist (gastroenterologist) who performs the test has dwindled to about $500/procedure (a procedure that takes about twenty minutes of time), the actual cost to insurance for a colonoscopy is often over $5000, with wide regional variation. Colonoscopies are billed as surgeries, allowing doctors to charge Medicare for many "incidental" fees that dramatically hike their reimbursement. They also employ anesthesiologists in their surgical suites, something done nowhere else in the world and that has been shown to be unnecessary, but which further escalates the cost. According to the article, anesthesiologists alone earn $1.1 billion each year from providing the unnecessary service.[265]

The lay press, both TV and print, recently lambasted the 2013 government sequester for denying older people necessary chemotherapy. In the sequester all doctors received a 2 percent cut in our Medicare reimbursement, one of many cuts we will be forced to swallow in the coming years. However, several intravenous infusion centers that administer chemotherapy stated publically that the cut would prevent them from offering chemotherapy to the elderly, with the assumption being that now those elderly would die from such blatant medical neglect. The press ran with the story, and the public ate it up. But no one thought to ask a few important questions. First, were these elderly patients really in need of intensive intravenous chemotherapy? Second, how much were these infusions centers and their specialist doctors earning that a 2 percent cut in reimbursement would financially ruin them?

This history of chemotherapy is a cloudy one, and one I do not have time to explore in this book. Suffice it to say that cancer specialists had until recently been paid very well to administer intravenous chemotherapy in their offices rather than prescribing oral treatment. In fact, when oral pills were given, the oncologists not only lost the huge markup they received on the intravenous drugs, but patients now had to pay for medicine; Medicare paid for expensive intravenous treatment but not for cheaper pills.[266][267] Of course, most patients believe that intensive intravenous treatment is stronger and more effective than pills anyway, so they appreciated the thorough care that the oncologists were rendering. The truth of that statement clearly strays from reality,[268] but in our specialized society truth rarely is powerful enough to trump perception. When Medicare stopped paying doctors directly for intravenous chemotherapy, the proportion of treatment being given as pills increased.[269][270] Now, though, infusion centers are paid to give the drugs, and they have an incentive to treat intravenously. Whether the 2 percent sequester cut truly prevented elderly patients from receiving "necessary" medicine is questionable, but the fact that the press did not ask those questions demonstrates the power and penetration of thorough care in our specialized medical world.

## The Dearth of Primary Care

Unfortunately for our eighty-five year old patients, society is inundated with specialized care and with specialists, while there are a dwindling number of generalists willing to take care of them. America has it backward with regard to specialists. I have read that in an ideal medical society there should be at least 50 percent generalists. In this country only 30 percent of doctors practice primary care and the rest are specialists.[271] These numbers continue to dwindle. We train many more specialists than primary care physicians, and a certain assumption prevails among doctors in training and society at large that specialists sit on a higher perch of the physician ladder than do primary care doctors. To many of my patients, and their families, my job as the primary care doctor is to coordinate their specialty care, to be a unifying presence. In other words, I exist not to render medical treatment, but rather to oversee the compartmentalized and intensive care that is being conducted within a specialized health care delivery system.

I remember when I interviewed at a large New York City hospital for medical school with the dean of admissions and I told him that my interest was in primary care. He said that a school like his did not train primary care doctors, because any school can train primary care doctors. At elite institutions they train specialists. I fought with him about it, and argued that his school should be ashamed of itself for not producing the type of doctor most needed in the country, whose job was the most intellectually difficult, even citing the fact that his hospital's own impoverished neighborhood was neglected by the institution because of its specialized mindset. By the time I returned back to college a week later, the dean's rejection letter was already in my mailbox. Even the medical school I did attend, which had a reputation for taking care of its impoverished neighborhood, and which produced some of the most prolific primary care thinkers in the world, sent the vast majority of its graduates to specialist programs.

The result of this trend is a dearth of primary care physicians and an abundance of specialists. In the medical worlds I have traversed, there seem to be as many cardiologists as internists, and they follow stable patients for simple problems several times a year. They perform procedures such as stress tests and echocardiograms regularly for screening, and control numbers (blood pressure, cholesterol) very tightly.

Endocrinologists follow simple diabetics, nephrologists (kidney doctors) follow patients with mild and asymptomatic kidney diseases, neurologists follow patients with stable dementia, and orthopedists follow people with simple arthritis. In all of these cases the specialists perform more tests, control numbers more tightly, and have more of a need to fix problems relevant to their field than do primary care doctors.[272] When a squadron of specialists follows my patients regularly, I lose control of much of their medical care. But there simply are not enough primary care doctors out there, so specialty care becomes the norm.

## Medical Training and Specialization

Why do so many medical students become specialists? The answer is multifold. First, since so many patients see specialists regularly and are allowed to do so by Medicare and other insurances, there is plenty of work for specialists, and there are more than enough specialty training slots open. Second, since specialty fields are procedure oriented, they are better remunerated and have more of a narrow focus, which is appealing. Many students graduate with tremendous debt and seek a good income, fearing that primary care salaries will be inadequate to pay back the debt and allow for a decent lifestyle. Third, at least in the view of students, specialists have a more interesting life than general doctors and carry more prestige. Fourth, in the course of their training, students and residents are exposed much more to specialty care than to primary care, since primary care doctors are less likely to be working in hospitals. Even when primary care doctors do interact with medical students and residents, they are academic doctors, not the type of doctor who most students and residents would ultimately become; there is minimal exposure to purely clinical primary care physicians. Fifth, many of the patients who students and residents see in the hospital during the course of their training are either "interesting cases" with highly complex specialty needs, or "boring cases" such as old nursing home patients who were dumped in the hospital for custodial care, the latter being perceived as the purview of the primary care physicians who had cared for them in the outside.

The dwindling supply of students and residents pursing primary care has significant ramifications for the health of our elderly and in the survivability of Medicare. In US medical schools, substantially fewer students retain interest in primary care fields compared to what they originally stated at the start of their schooling.[273] Even worse, only about 20 percent of students actually pursue a primary care field by the end of their training. That compares to 54 percent of students who entered primary care in 1998.[274] Medical schools, which do very little to encourage students to enter primary care, consistently try to exaggerate how many potential primary care doctors they train[275] without actually encouraging their students to enter primary care. Primary care residency slots remain unfilled more than others, they have the highest level of dissatisfaction among students, and they have a perceived lack of prestige.[276] [277] [278] Therefore, it is no surprise that we have a primary care shortage in this country. The number of doctors who practice primary care dropped from 59 percent in 1949 to 37 percent in 1998,[279] and that number continues to decline. With the many costly and time-consuming reforms being thrust on the laps of primary care doctors by the ACA and Medicare, many practicing doctors are either retiring, refusing to accept Medicare, or are becoming concierge practices that take no insurance at all. This is only exacerbating our primary care shortage, and it is likely to get worse.

In my own experience as a medical student and medical resident, I had the fortune to be exposed to a wealth of wonderful primary care thinkers. But in New York most of the students turned their backs on primary care fields, and very few of us pursued that route. Even those who accepted residencies in internal medicine explicitly stated that they intended to seek further training as cardiologists or gastroenterologists, two of the most highly reimbursed specialties at the time. My residency training was unique in that many primary care thinkers taught us, but even there less than a third of our class left training to practice primary care, a number that is far higher than the national average. According to the doctors who still work in that hospital training center, only a handful enter primary care now. I remember in our first week of residency a fellow resident approached me and my wife. She asked us what we were planning to do after training. I told her primary care, and she smirked. My wife told her maybe something like gastroenterology or endocrinology. The girl smiled at my wife, "Good for you," she said. "Those are much better choices." That girl became our chief resident and ultimately a cardiologist, and her view is very common among those who train in my field. Most think you have to be insane to become a primary care doctor. Both my wife and I practice primary care, and we enjoy our jobs immensely. But without a doubt we are among the few who still would enter primary care if given the choice today.

Primary care doctors earn far less than specialists. The salary discrepancy in medical fields is not something that is determined by the free market. If that were the case, why would anesthesiologists make substantially more money than some surgeons who actually operate?[280] Patients spend time and effort to pick out their surgeons, and the ultimate outcome of their operation is largely in their surgeon's hands. Anesthesiologists certainly play an important role in the surgery, as do nurses and other ancillary staff, but patients do not chose them or even give much thought to what they do. In the free market, they likely would pay a surgeon far more than an anesthesiologist. In most cases, patients do not have any impact on or knowledge of what any of their doctors earn.

The choice of what a doctor earns is in the hands of CMS. Medicare sets rates, and then most other insurances follow suit. If I earn $100 to see a patient in the office and a cardiologist earns $150 for a visit and a dermatologist earns $200 to cut off a mole, those charges are dictated directly by CMS. We as physicians cannot charge any more or less than what CMS dictates, and patient preference has no role.

At a recent AMDA conference we heard a talk by Paul McGann from CMS about new changes in Medicare, and several people in the audience asked why CMS did not work harder to achieve some reimbursement parity among doctors. He told us that in fact CMS had delegated reimbursement rates to the AMA (American Medical Association) as a way of appeasing doctors, and it was that agency that had not done anything to ameliorate the salary divergence.[281] The relative value scale update committee (RUC) is a thirty-one-physician committee in the AMA that recommends what CMS will pay for visits and procedures. The committee is specialist dominated, and thus primary care doctors have little voice.[282] The committee meets every year to derive income formulas, basing much of its calculation on estimates of how much physician time a procedure or visit requires. But, as the *Washington Post* revealed, those time estimates are greatly exaggerated for specialty procedures. Also, since the members of the committee are largely appointed by specialist societies, "the problem arises from giving the AMA and specialty societies too much influence over physician pay."[283] Given that only a minority of doctors belong to the AMA, and that virtually no primary care doctors are part of that organization, it is not surprising that it has done nothing to fix this crucial problem. What is surprising is that CMS, which is incessantly trumpeting the need for more primary care doctors in any sensible medical reform model, has done nothing to remedy the ultimate barrier to people actually pursuing primary care fields: pay inequity. By one report anesthesiologists earn approximately $309,000, cardiologists $314,000, orthopedists $315,000, gastroenterologists $303,000, oncologists $295,000, and primary care internists (my field) $166,000 (see footnote 23). By the estimates of the *Washington Post* article (which seem to slant the salaries up a bit) the average orthopedist earns $520,000, gastroenterologists $480,000, ophthalmologists $354,000, and primary care internists $215,000. In either calculation, primary care doctors are earning approximately half of other specialists. CMS has given primary care doctors a 10 percent bonus on all Medicare billing for the past few years, but that will not likely persist, as most of its other incentives have turned into disincentives within a few years, and that is a paltry increase that does not come close to narrowing the income gap between primary care doctors and specialists.

Because primary care doctors do not have a lobbying organization, while most other specialties do, no one is pushing very hard to create an environment in primary care that would attract new recruits. That is why there is no perceivable end to our specialized society. Even if Medicare changed its rules and dissuaded older patients from following a specialized path in pursuit of their health, there simply would not be enough primary care doctors around to take up the slack.

## The Problem with Heightened Expectations in a Specialized Society

Heightened expectations often drive specialized care, because many patients believe that thorough diagnosis and treatment is the best way to attack and defeat medical decline. There is hardly a patient who has received a stent who does not credit his cardiologist for saving his life, proclaiming that no other course of care would have saved him. Patients are similarly indebted to the endocrinologist who treats their diabetes, or the neurologist who put them on the life-saving Alzheimer's drug after conducting thorough testing, or the nephrologist who is keeping a close eye on their kidney function and repairing every possible errant number that if left unchecked would kill them, or even who puts them on dialysis.

But when expectations escalate, then poor outcomes are viewed not as part of the inevitable decline in aging, but rather as a failure. People become obsessed with looking for and fixing everything, something they have come to believe is achievable. That is the natural consequence of our specialized society. Unlike in the case of Mrs. A., who I described in the introduction, the success of medical intervention is no longer measured by happiness and quality, but rather by tests and numbers and life expectancy. Mom may be happy, but she is not well, her medical conditions are not adequately controlled, and we are going to do whatever it takes to ascertain why. And when mom declines further, we all wonder how that can possibly happen, even as experts repair one leak after another in her fragile body, when they fix her numbers and order more tests. The problem is never viewed as being related to aging itself, or even ascribed to the faulty repair work being done, but rather to even more fixable problems that are amenable to still more repairs as long as we fight hard enough to identify the salient issues. Specialization does not accept defeat. Specialization pushes everyone to keep digging deeper into elderly bodies, keep pouring in drugs and tests, keep monitoring every possible number, without any regard to quality. It is the very antithesis of a palliative approach to care. And it leads to an expectation that adverse outcomes are not acceptable.

I found it fascinating that in my ACO, which is a new Medicare program that we will discuss later designed to save money, one of the quality indicators on which I will be graded, and on which my monetary bonus may be calculated, is access of my Medicare patients to specialists. Even as they innovate to cut costs and provide quality care, Medicare is rewarding doctors who encourage their elderly patients to pursue specialized care. Medicare does not seem concerned that our specialized medical society may be having an adverse impact on the health of older Americans and on the rapidly increasing cost of care. Somehow, it has missed the boat on that one.

## Lawyers

One untoward consequence of our specialized society and its heightened expectations is a belief by Americans in the invincibility of the health care delivery system. If an illness is not cured, if an untoward medical outcome occurs, if the perils of aging cannot be reversed, then certainly someone has to be at fault. After all, with so much technology, so many promises, such well-trained experts who have the most advanced tools at their disposal, why should any of our older citizens have to endure medical declines? When bad outcomes do occur, often a finger is pointed and someone is blamed. Such thinking is what triggers the fear of malpractice among many in the medical community, a fear that instigates a posture of defensive medicine leading to even more aggressive care and higher societal costs.

Is malpractice really as bad as doctors think? My father, who is a lawyer, often debunks the myth of malpractice. He claims that no lawyer in his right mind would take a case that does not have merit, because the cost of researching and litigating such a case would far exceed any potential payment. Much of the literature would agree.[284] [285] [286]

And yet, malpractice, or the fear of malpractice, impacts everything we do. Not just what we do as doctors, but what patients think. How facilities and nurses act. And how families interact with the medical system. As long as malpractice remains an incessant threat, it will be an excuse used by everyone in the medical establishment to pursue a course of aggressive medical care.[287] [288] [289] The line that "I'm ordering those tests so I'm not sued" is uttered regularly from the mouths of doctors. Even when not spoken, it is often thought.

Several studies have demonstrated a correlation between the degree of malpractice fear experienced by a doctor and his/her likelihood of ordering more tests and procedures.[290] [291] The same phenomenon occurs too when physicians have read about a lawsuit or know of doctors who are sued.[292] Such "defensive medicine" leads doctors to practice aggressive medical care despite the fact that they know other more conservative approaches are medically acceptable.[293] Given that in a typical forty-year career of a physician he/she will be involved with an open, unresolved malpractice claim 11 percent of the time, which amounts to 50.7 months on average,[294] and given that most doctors often know someone being sued or have read about high profile cases, the threat of legal action, whether real or imagined, sits heavily on us when we make clinical decisions. And while studies suggest that the threat of malpractice itself does not diminish quality of care,[295] the fear of malpractice certainly exacerbates a costly and dangerous medical ethos that further promotes a "thorough" approach to care.

Who could think otherwise given the omnipresent threat of suit? The TVs are flooded by commercials showing shady lawyers pleading for you to call them if you have any adverse outcomes. It may be birth trauma. It may be a symptom that was missed. It may be related to using a particular drug or not diagnosing a condition. Or it may be the vague crime of nursing home negligence, as we will discuss later.

My father and I have talked often about whether malpractice reform will really improve the environment of aggressive care. I believe that if you dismantle the allure of "pain and suffering" rewards, then very few people will sue. There simply will not be enough of a potential financial reward to pay off all parties, especially in geriatric cases. And in my opinion, pain and suffering should not be compensated by giving someone money. If doctors or facilities are negligent, then they should be judged by their peers, and an appropriate punishment should be implemented.

"Let's face it, "my father said. "Even with pain and suffering, there is not any incentive to take a case that is not legitimate. No lawyer would do that. Not for an old person."

And then, soon after he made that statement, I was sued.

During my office hours an official appearing person (I thought he was a policeman) stood outside of my exam room door. When I walked out, he handed me a letter. "Dr. Lazris, I am serving you with a summons." It was one of the most demeaning and frightening moments of my professional career. I could only wonder what I may have done. Many possible incidents flooded my brain. Meanwhile, the patients standing in the office peered at me as though I had done something very wrong. Word soon trickled to my other patients too. Dr. Lazris was served a summons.

I made a few calls and was given the number of a lawyer, who I was told would be representing me. I was also given the name of the patient whose daughter was pressing charges. It had actually been one of my favorite patients, and she had a daughter with whom I got along well. She was ninety-eight years old, had moved to the nursing home where I worked because of worsening dementia, frailty, and poor balance, and then had moved to another nursing home facility for reasons that

I believed were due to her being too far from her daughter, and at that point I lost contact with her. She did very well in the original nursing home, but her daughter did not like it at all. She was very upset about losing control over her mom's care. She felt her mom was not given enough attention, was not given her medicines properly, and was treated with neglect. She complained to me about it several times, and on each occasion I did what I could to help alleviate the daughter's fears. In fact, despite her daughter's concerns, my patient thrived in the nursing home, and was typically very happy and healthy.

I requested her chart from medical records, and I dug though it for many hours. I still could not conceive of what I had done wrong. My lawyer called, and offered only vague answers. He was pleasant, and he said I should not worry. We set up a time to meet in about a week. I canceled all my patients for that day, the first of many times I would have to halt my clinical duties to pursue this frustrating case.

I traveled to Baltimore and ascended a large building to a beautiful office high above the city. There I met with my lawyer. He then elucidated the case to me. Apparently the patient had developed a cough. She was treated with Robitussin by a nurse practitioner who worked at the nursing home, although not as my employee. A few days after that, the patient's cough had not resolved, although she was otherwise well. The nurse practitioner then started antibiotics. The patient became weak for a few days and ate poorly. At some point during this period the daughter had called me, and I saw the patient. By that time she was recovering, and soon after was her usual self. But the daughter claimed that delay in treatment for bronchitis had caused her mom to decline to the point that she was now dependent on a wheelchair.

I looked at my lawyer, both confused and scared. There was no case here. Nothing went wrong. This was a ninety-eight-year-old woman who was treated properly for a common infection. She had no adverse outcome. In fact, I later learned that she lived to almost a hundred. "This can't be serious," I said to him. "I mean, we can just dismiss this nonsense, right?"

"It doesn't work that way."

"Well, I'll tell you, I refuse to settle. Nothing was done wrong. I'll fight this as far as I have to to clear my name."

The lawyer laughed. "Don't worry. Luckily this happened in Baltimore County. If it had happened a few miles down the road in Baltimore City, it would be a different matter. Baltimore City jurors always rule for the plaintiff. They view malpractice cases as though they are a lottery. But juries in the County are more reasonable. They'll need a very solid case to take this to court. I'm not worried. We just can't get emotional. Stick to the facts. Do your homework."

My lawyer then informed me that an expert witness—a doctor who worked in the town where I now practice—had reviewed the case and found that there were indeed issues of negligence in the patient's care. Since that day I have learned a lot about "experts," doctors who are hired by lawyers to determine the merit of a case. I have read books about experts, and I have friends who earn a portion of their income working with lawyers. I have seen "experts" from the great bastions of medical science, and from the lowest rungs of medical practice, twist a case to make it fit nicely for the lawyer.

Expert physicians get paid very well, much better than they would if they practiced medicine. They do their work at home, and tell the lawyer how many hours they work, including the hours engaged in thought. When they find evidence that helps their lawyer's case, they are given more work by the lawyer. When they find less merit in a case, it is unlikely they will get more work from that lawyer. So all the incentive for these "experts" is to agree with the lawyer's case and find evidence to support it.[296]

Without physician experts, there would be no significant threat of malpractice. The "expert witness for hire" business is a lucrative and thriving industry among physicians. Many doctors advertise their services in legal magazines, many obtain a large portion of their income from helping lawyers.[297] No expert has to ground his/her claims in the concrete block of truth or standard of care. Some provide "dishonest or medically unjustified testimony due largely to the lucrative nature of expert testimony." Judges do not balk at such practice; they allow all testimony in their courts, leaving it to the plaintiff's "expert" to debunk the defense's "expert," and for the jury to ascertain which expert's claims are legitimate.[298] Of course, when a doctor is fed large sums of money to help a lawyer's case, and when that doctor knows that the ability to be hired for subsequent cases may be contingent on his/her ability to make the lawyer happy, then there is "potential for physician experts to fuel inappropriate litigation through testimony that is not well grounded in prevailing clinical standards or science."[299] Before we blame lawyers for our malpractice mess, it may be best for the medical profession to look at itself in the mirror.

For me, my case continued forward. I went for depositions, taking more time off from work. There I met the daughter's lawyer, who sat with a smirk on his facing wearing a Hawaiian shirt. Although my lawyer had called him a lightweight, I was taken aback by how cordial they were to each other. I realized that without the schlock lawyer wearing a Hawaiian shirt and having a bunch of paid-off "experts" at his disposal, my lawyer would not be able to get cases. Both of them profited from the current system, even if my lawyer stood on the right side of the law, as least as I perceived things.

"Stay calm," my lawyer told me. "Just answer questions simply and calmly. If you don't know, say so."

I really did not need his help. This case was not very difficult for me to defend. I sat at a big table with both lawyers there, and a third lawyer as well, the nursing home's lawyer, who was there for reasons unclear to me at the time.

The depositions were actually among the most enjoyable hours I have ever spent. I stayed calm. I stuck to my points. I shredded every claim made by the "expert." I explained what we did to care for the patient and why the patient received appropriate geriatric care. The Hawaiian shirt lawyer constantly tried to bait me, pushing me into saying something bad about the nursing home where my patient had lived. I never fell for his chicanery. But I now understood why the nursing home's lawyer was at the table.

After the deposition was over my lawyer took me into his office and shook my hand. "Good job," he told me.

"So does that end it?" I asked. "They clearly don't have a case."

"It's not that simple," he said.

I paused. "It seems to me that the only reason they are suing me is to get to the nursing home. Could that be true?"

My lawyer just nodded yes. He explained that when someone sues a facility they typically name anyone involved, hoping the other defendants will try to save themselves by denouncing the facility. It is all a very ugly game.

For me, the cost in time and anxiety was piled on high, as well as the cost to a system that had to hire my lawyer to defend me, and a cost that helped feed everything I knew was wrong with our medical system.

The case continued. Letters back and forth. More accusations for me to challenge. And then something happened, something that shocked me more than anything else that transpired during this case, and something that ended the case for good.

My lawyer called me. He told me that the patient's daughter just had her deposition, the very daughter who brought the case against me. And in the deposition she said that the only good thing that happened during her mother's time at the nursing home was her relationship with Dr. Lazris. She made it very clear that I had done nothing wrong.

"That has to end this case!" I insisted to my lawyer.

And in fact, by that afternoon, the case against me was dismissed.

Still, to this day, the case haunts me. Not that it replays in my mind, although it does do that, only to remind me just how broken the system is. But more pragmatically, there is not an application to an insurance company or to a hospital or to a license that I fill out in which I do not have to indicate that I was sued and then provide a separate explanation about what transpired. It is though I am scarred by the suit, and I will be for the rest of my professional career. Even though the frivolous case was dismissed, it hangs over me and causes me endless inconvenience and embarrassment.

I always wonder about how I would feel if I were sued multiple times by people who find willing lawyers and experts and hope to win the lottery. So many doctors are, or are at least threatened. All of us watch the commercials, or hear about accusations thrown at us, and we wonder if we are next.

To debate the soundness of my father's perception of malpractice—that its impact is far less than what people think—against the malpractice obsession that suffocates the medical community is irrelevant and pointless. The fact remains that as long as malpractice hovers as a threat, it will impact behavior. As with the dogma of specialization that fuels it, malpractice breeds a culture of aggressive care and heightened expectation that is both counterproductive to older patients and very expensive. The logical assumption ingrained in this culture is that older patients who are deteriorating deserve the most excessive care possible in an effort to save them. Such a belief often sends patients to the ultimate bastion of aggressive, specialized, and thorough care that exists in our country: the hospital. It is that chapter we will explore next.

# 4

# HOSPITALIZATION, THE PINNACLE OF THOROUGH

*"Most people die in hospitals, tied up with tubes and with their*
*bodies pumped full of drugs. Yet most would rather die at home and*
*with more control over the timing and manner of their death."*
Geoff Mulgan, CEO National Endowment
of Science Technology and the Arts

The ultimate result of specialization, of the need to thoroughly defeat aging by righting every unearthed ailment and flooding the body
with pills, tests, and procedures, is hospitalization. If specialty care
is needed to address each problem that arises, then hospital level of
care is necessary when those problems become severe. In the hospital,
patients can receive intensive treatment, all the necessary tests and
procedures, the strongest medicines, and access to every form of specialty care. Hospitals have saved many of my oldest patients at some
point in their lives. Just ask them or their families, and they will tell
you. Recently I had a patient tell me that if he had come to the hospital
only ten minutes later he would have been dead. These are common
tales I hear every day. They are visions of hospital care shared by patients, doctors, and society at large. But if we explore why Medicare
is failing, and to where a large chunk of its expenses are evaporating

without improved outcome, we do not have to look much beyond the hospital.[300]

Especially at a point of desperation, many elderly people and their families, as well as their doctors, believe that only a hospital can provide the needed care to bring a very sick person back from the brink of drastic decline. What we will show is that in fact hospitals frequently instigate more harm in the elderly than actually providing benefit. But more significantly, the hospital is perceived as a beacon of care not only because of what it is felt to provide, but rather because no other options exist. As we discussed, Medicare's inception in 1965 came with a caveat designed to appease the AMA: The hospital would remain predominant in the spectrum of care. Very few regulations hampered hospital care, and in fact hospitalized care fell under the umbrella of Medicare A, an insurance given to all elderly and disabled people without charge. Medicare pays for hospitals, and because Medicare A is typically easier to access and more generous in its allocation of resources than Medicare B, the hospital is often the least expensive destination for ill patients.

Four million Americans have Part A only, which represents 6 percent of all Medicare beneficiaries. Part A requires patients to pay an $1184 deductible, after which all services are covered for the first sixty days.[301] People with only Part A have no choice but to travel to the hospital for all of their care. Part B covers most expenses other than medications. In Part B there is a much lower deductible, but there is a 20 percent copay associated with tests and visits. Ninety percent of elderly Americans also carry a supplemental insurance plan that pays for the hospital deductible and for the 20 percent that Medicare B does not cover, thus making most medical care free after their premiums are paid.[302] The small percentage of people with Part B and no supplemental insurance likely will find hospital care less expensive to them than care at home, especially if they need many tests and procedures. But even for those with supplemental insurance, Medicare's rules and its payment system frequently push reluctant patients into the hospital. The hospital is a conundrum of good and bad, especially for our oldest patients; frequently the elderly are tossed there for poorly conceived reasons or out of financial necessity, and often the end result is poor outcome at high cost.

## Medication Errors

As a medical student in New York I worked with resident doctors, who, in teaching hospitals, essentially manage all facets of patient care. A few days before Thanksgiving, when we were all trying to devise strategies to get out early and spend some time at home, our team was caring for two women, both with similar last names. One had diabetes, the other did not. The diabetic woman was old and demented, but her big smile and frequent hilarious one-liners kept us all in stitches. The other woman was fairly ill with a drug related infection. One day we received an urgent lab result that one of the women's sugars had shot up to 600, a very high value. The resident instructed me to give the young woman insulin and to recheck the sugar in a few hours. But when we did check it the next morning, it remained high, and the young woman looked even sicker than before. We then checked a finger stick sugar, and it showed a very low sugar number, prompting us to give the young woman an infusion of sugar water into her veins. We thought that there was a lab error, and pushed it aside. The next day on routine labs, we again received notice of a high sugar, this time over 800. Again we checked a finger stick sugar, and it was now normal. A few days passed, and we then saw another sugar, this time it was 1200. Suddenly my resident realized what was going on. The labs were actually from the older, demented woman whose name was virtually identical to the younger woman. When we ran to see her and checked her finger stick sugar, it was off the charts. She was as happy as can be, and I remember to this day what she said: "Why are all of you coming into the barber shop now? You know I'm next in line. But if you're in a rush, you can go ahead. It's no trouble for me." She died a few hours later, likely from hyperglycemia. But what transpired subsequently inflicted a permanent scar on my medical psyche. As we all feared the consequences of our mistake, the patient's brother came to the hospital bearing a large box of candies. He handed the box to us. "Thank you so much for taking care of my sister," he said with a tear in his eye. "I know she was too sick to be saved by you people, but you gave her the best care she could have got, and the family appreciates all that you did for her." We said nothing. In retrospect, we easily could have killed both of the patients with our mistake. But instead of a reprimand, we received candy and a hug.

Throughout my days working in hospitals, rushing through patients about whom I knew very little, paging through lists of medicines and tests and numbers, I did my best to keep on top of all medical issues that emerged. But I cannot even begin to relay how often the wrong medicines were given (such as Dilantin, a seizure medicine, instead of Diltiazem, a blood pressure medicine), important medicines were overlooked and not given, or even another patient's entire medicine list was inadvertently substituted for my patient's list because of a clerical error, leading my patient to be on completely erroneous drugs, some of which could have been lethal, and to not be on his usual drugs, some of which may have been necessary. I have had patients whose blood pressures plummeted and who were sent to an Intensive Care Unit (ICU) and given the million dollar work-up in search of infection or heart dysfunction, only to find out that they were accidently put on blood pressure medicines that they had not taken at home. Sometimes the lists of medicines were derived from past hospital stays, other times they were written down after talking to a family member or a confused patient, sometimes they came from a fax sent by the doctor's office that itself was either barely legible or not accurate. Regardless, hospital medication error is something with which we contend that is dangerous and difficult to avoid.

Medical mistakes are common in the hospital, especially among the elderly who are often taking many medicines. Such mistakes instigate tremendous morbidity and mortality, making hospital errors the eighth leading cause of death in the country. Each year, 1.3 million hospitalized patients suffer a serious complication from a medical error.[303] [304]

Errors occur commonly on hospital admission, but even on discharge errors occur with similar surprising frequency. As we will discuss, during transitions of patients from a hospital to a nursing home, a likely destination for many of the very old patients in our Medicare community, medicine lists often are severely mangled and it can require days or weeks to repair the errors and to fix any damage that may have been incurred.

## The Sting of Aggression

Often hospital "mistakes" are of a more insidious nature, resulting from the adrenaline driven atmosphere that exists within hospital walls. From the time I was a medical student, through my days ward attending in a teaching hospital, I witnessed the deluge of aggression that greets those who enter a hospital's hallowed halls. I remember one day as an attending I came in and noted that most of my patients were being seen by multiple specialists, all of whom were ordering their own tests and paying close attention to their own organs of interest. I questioned the medical resident, and he told me that as a teaching hospital resident he felt obligated to have specialists take care of the many chronic problems each patient had, even if the problems were quiescent. Not only did he believe such care to be superior, but also he thought it would be educational for the residents on each of the specialty teams to put their hands into the care. How else would they learn?

Even later in my career, I often called in specialists to ease my burden. If a patient was too sick, or I received too many calls from nurses during the day, I made sure to have a cardiologist, a pulmonologist, an infectious disease expert, and even a surgeon look in on my patients to deflect some of my own responsibility. Today I see hospitalist doctors doing the same thing. Hospitalists are doctors hired by the hospital to take care of hospitalized patients, since most of us in primary care are unable logistically to care for our own patients in the hospital. Many hospitalists are very young, just out of residency, with little experience behind them.

They do not know their patients well, and in my own estimation very few whom I have encountered are cognizant of how to care for the elderly. Typically they call in a squadron of specialists, tackling one problem at a time. The end result is specialized, aggressive care.

Mrs. R. went to the hospital for a rapid heartbeat. I usually treat that in my office, and order a little home health so a nurse can keep an eye on the situation, but the cardiologist wanted her in the hospital, and she could not really afford home health aides (which are not paid for by Medicare, while the far more expensive hospital stay is), so there she went. Once there they found she had a little fluid on her lung, so they gave her an intravenous diuretic called Lasix. But they gave her too much. She starting peeing everywhere and getting upset. She also became dehydrated and her blood electrolytes destabilized. Nurses incessantly invaded her room at all hours to draw blood and check vital signs as they carried on conversations outside of her room. She started getting delirious. They tied her down and gave her medicine to calm her. She thrashed all the more. Her kidney function worsened from the powerful medications and her inability to eat. They pushed food and fluids on her, and she inadvertently sucked some of the food into her lungs. She developed a raging pneumonia, requiring her to be intubated and hooked up to a breathing machine in an intensive care unit. There she lost blood, developed complications from antibiotics including excessive diarrhea, and required even more aggressive care. She lasted two weeks in the ICU before dying, probably at a cost of over $100,000 paid by Medicare for an outcome that did not have to occur.

Very often my older patients are physically tied down in the hospital, are subjected to toxic medicines to calm them down, and become delirious. These are not necessarily people who are ever confused when they are well, but the trauma of the hospital induces it. I remember coming to a medical floor one day to find one of my favorite patients tied down to his bed. He was thrashing and yelling in a way I could have never imagined. I untied him. He had a Foley catheter in his bladder and two

IV lines in his arms. I told the nurses to remove all of that and to send him home. They thought I was insane. But within an hour of his arrival home, with his daughter staying with him that night, he was himself again. Hospital delirium is common in the elderly, and the outcomes are not good. Many patients lose function from their delirium and are more likely to develop dementia or have worsening memory subsequent to their hospital stay.[305] [306]

Mrs. G. fell and broke her shoulder. She was already frail, and could not function on her own with a broken shoulder. Ideally she needed either a few hours a day of home health, or a short stay in a rehab unit, both of which were cheap and safe options but not ones she could afford under current Medicare rules. So she went to the hospital, where admission was easily justified by her other medical conditions, some of which had become worse since the fall, including higher blood pressure and a little dehydration. Not only would Medicare pay for the hospital stay, but it would pay for up to a three-month rehabilitation stay after the hospitalization, something she and her daughter felt would be necessary before she could return home. For her to qualify for rehabilitation to be paid, though, Mrs. G. had to stay in the hospital for at least three nights, something that is a very strict Medicare rule. So we agreed to prolong her hospital stay for her to qualify, something we labeled as "punching our patient's ticket," meaning that we were helping our patients to save some money by keeping them in for three nights. Mrs. G. ultimately did make it to the rehab center, but weeks later, and at a high personal and financial cost. Her hospital stay nearly destroyed her. She was given too much pain medicine, developing severe constipation and bowel dysfunction, then a urine infection from her catheter, then diarrhea from the antibiotic used to treat the urine infection and the medicine used to treat her prior constipation, then delirium, and inability to eat, and the need for intravenous fluids, and infections from the intravenous needle sites, and fluid overload, and anemia requiring transfusions, and complications from the transfusions. A half dozen specialists followed her, and she was exposed to tests nearly every day. She had a very thorough hospital stay. I hardly remember all the details, other than how terrible it was. One problem led to another, one treatment to another disaster, until she became a shadow of herself. Medicare did pay for her stay at the hospital and then at the rehabilitation unit, which is all she had wanted, but at a cost of probably a hundred thousand dollars and my patient's soul and vitality.

Mrs. G.'s story is not at all atypical. Older people in the hospital do not fare well. Their bodies are fragile, and treating one problem often instigates another. In the hospital patients are assaulted by aggressive doctors and nurses of every stripe, many of whom are not addressing the problem that brought the patient to the hospital but rather problems that were "discovered" while at the hospital. That leads to more tests, medicines, treatments, and ultimately to more stress, confusion, and complications. And those complications lead to more interventions, which lead to more complications, and so on, until the cascade of failure takes on a life of its own.

A copious number of studies demonstrate the poor outcomes incurred by hospitalizing elderly people, especially those who are frail and demented. The mortality of older adults sent to the hospital is high, both during hospitalization and in the immediate post-hospital period. A quarter of hospitalized elders sent from a hospital to a rehabilitation unit are dead within six months despite the enormous resources thrust at them. Long-term outcomes are much worse.[307] [308] [309] Those hospitalized with advanced dementia have a very high short-term mortality, especially when artificially fed.[310] In one of the most common conditions for which the elderly are hospitalized, congestive heart failure, the one-year outcome is abysmal, and the cost of thorough care does not translate into any meaningful results.[311]

Hospitalized elders have significant functional loss after a hospital stay, especially if they become confused in the hospital. This is most pronounced among our frailest elderly and those with dementia.[312] Hospitalization leads to decreased muscle tone, decreased nutritional integrity, and an increase in both urinary incontinence and skin breakdown. Restriction of activity in the hospital accounts for much of this decline, but so too does the cascade of aggressive care that the hospital floods upon their oldest patients. Much of the functional loss is irreversible.[313] [314] [315]

# Infections

The hospital itself is a brewing caldron of resistant bacteria that can cause terrible infections, even for those who only reach the emergency room.[316] Many of my patients emerge with infections that disable them or take their lives after a hospital stay. It is estimated that preventable infections account for 75,000 deaths a year[317] and mistakes in the hospital account for 200,000 deaths a year.[318] It is felt that more than 200 people die of hospital acquired infections daily, which is as though a plane crashes every day and kills everyone on board. Even one plane crash is front page news for weeks. Deaths from hospital infections, which occur every day, are barely noticed.

My older, frail patients are particularly vulnerable to the sting of hospital acquired infections. So many return home or to their long-term care facilities with massive bouts of diarrhea caused by cdiff, a virulent colon bacteria that profligates in hospitals and overwhelms the bowels of many older patients, especially if they were exposed to broad spectrum antibiotics in the hospital. These patients become dehydrated quickly, get confused, develop nutritional depletion, and have significant derangements in their body chemistry. Their functional status declines rapidly and they are unable to participate in rehabilitation. Skin breakdown is common. They are often isolated in their rooms and are unable to leave, being greeted by nurses and doctors wearing gowns and masks, as they sit in a pile of liquid, putrid stool. Cdiff is a consequence not only of a hospital stay, but also of even an emergency room visit. We treat it with even more antibiotics, sometimes for weeks, sometimes unsuccessfully. Patients die of cdiff. They physically and mentally decline. And it is more common than people realize.

My patients also return with other resistant bugs such as MRSA, E. coli, and Klebsiella. These cause very difficult to treat skin infections, urinary tract infections, and even pneumonias. They too lead to decline, to more antibiotics, and to isolation. As these superbugs grow in the hospital and latch themselves to older bodies, they spread beyond the confines of the hospital walls. Like with so many hospital complications, infections occur after discharge and are thus not always ascribed to the hospital stay itself. But the hospital is their immediate cause, and their consequences can be devastating.

## The Benefits of Hospitalization?

Given how dangerous hospitals are for the elderly, and how common it is for the elderly to be admitted to hospitals in America, there must be very good reason for older patients to be hospitalized. It is common lore that when the elderly are too sick to be cared for at home, when they are met with changes in condition such as worsening memory or dizziness, when they develop serious infections such as pneumonia or potentially dangerous diseases such as heart failure and A-fib, then hospitals are the safest and most sensible places in which to get proper and thorough care. The truth, though, is much more dubious.

I have challenged many doctors to show me a single study that demonstrates the efficacy of hospitalization in the elderly for stroke, pneumonia, change in memory, fainting, small heart attacks, and a wide range of medical problems for which my older patients regularly are admitted. I am still waiting for a response. I have searched the medical literature and found nothing that convinces me of any significant clinical benefit of hospitalization for these conditions that would justify the risk.

In fact, studies show that elderly patients treated in their own beds do as well or better than those sent to the hospital. Pneumonia is a prime example. In patients who are in nursing homes or who are nursing home eligible, treatment within the facility or at home affords a better outcome with less functional decline than does treatment within the hospital. People die less, recover more quickly, and are not as prone to delirium as are hospitalized patients.[319] [320] [321] Even more significantly, they are able to stay with nurses and/or family who know them, are in a comfortable environment that is familiar, and are not subjected to the specialized assault that will likely greet them in the hospital.

A congestive heart failure (CHF) study further pounds this fact home. Very few diagnoses are more likely to lead to hospitalization than CHF, a condition where the heart is not functioning properly and the lungs can fill up with fluid. In the hospital such patients are diuresed with medicines that pull fluid out of their lungs. Of course, since they are in the hospital, they are often subjected to multiple tests, specialty visits, new (and often erroneous) medicines, and potential infections. Sometimes they are given too much diuresis sending them down a road of dehydration, excessive urination, and infection. Almost all of them have a urinary catheter shoved in their bladder and IV lines inserted into their arms, which are more foci of infection and potential delirium. But it is considered standard of care to hospitalize such patients; the only other option would be a more palliative approach whereby they stay at home and are kept comfortable. The basic assumption sewed into palliative care is that such patients, by eschewing aggressive interventions such as hospitalization, are accepting death as the alternative. But research demonstrates just the opposite. With CHF, people live an average of eighty-one days longer with a palliative approach than with standard treatment, including hospitalization. Many other severe illnesses are similarly better treated with palliative care then with aggressive care. In fact, in a Dartmouth study, full-dose palliative care produced better quality of life, decreased depression, and *increased survival* compared to a more standard, aggressive route.[322] Of course, palliative care not only is safer and more compassionate than hospitalization, but it is far less expensive to Medicare and to society.

People treated with a palliative approach are not simply neglected and left to die just because they are not pushed into a hospital and shoved down a bumpy road of thorough intervention. A palliative approach to CHF, for instance, would have as its goal patient comfort, which would therefore aim to reduce the shortness of breath associated with increased fluid retention. Such patients may weigh themselves regularly, be helped with medication and disease management by care coordinators, be offered dietary and exercise counseling, receive periodic visits by home health nurses and physical therapists, and have more regular appointments with their primary care doctor. The objective is to prevent any exacerbations that may lead to worsening CHF. Since most elderly prefer to stay at home, palliative services can deliver the bulk of their care in the home environment, especially if a patient is considered homebound. The fact that such an approach reflects what most patients request, is less expensive, and leads to better outcomes does not mean that it is feasible. Medicare pays for hospitalization and aggressive management far more than for any meaningful palliative home care, especially for those patients who may require more custodial help.

Many other ill patients would likely benefit by being treated with care and dignity at home instead of in a hospital. Syncope (passing out), strokes, increased confusion, and excessive fatigue are all symptoms that drive many of my patients to the hospital. There is no evidence that hospitalization improves outcomes in any of these conditions, and ample evidence that hospitalization in general is dangerous for elderly patients, as we have discussed. But the natural reflex action when someone faints or becomes confused or exhibits signs of stroke is to push them into a hospital. The latter situation is more nuanced, since obtaining a CT scan for potential stroke victims can help drive treatment depending on whether the patient has a true ischemic stroke or a bleed, but beyond that there is little that the hospital can do to ameliorate the damage done by a stroke in an elderly patient. In my experience, many elderly stroke patients are harmed by the hospital, whether by having their blood pressures pushed too low, or fed in a way that causes them to aspirate into their lungs, or given fluids and pushed into heart failure. They are also potential victims of resistant infections, medication errors, and hospital-induced delirium.

The one significant intervention that can potentially help stroke victims, and that pushes everyone to the hospital as quickly as possible, is TPA, or clot-busting medicine. Many of my patients or their families insist that they need to be hospitalized within hours of a potential stroke so they can receive the miracle medicines that dissolve blood clots. But in patients over eighty, according to a recent study, 16 percent of patients given TPA develop a significant brain bleed, and none of the patients who received TPA had improved function compared to standard care patients after three months.[323]

That is not to say that the hospital is an inappropriate place to go for catastrophic illness requiring intensive care treatment or emergent surgery. But even in those circumstances, in frail elderly patients who have dementia, the hospital may simply make the last days of someone's life more traumatic and extremely expensive. Much of end-of-life care occurs in the intensive care unit of a hospital, where expensive and traumatic care leads to no measurable medical benefit for the frail elderly patient.[324][325][326] A huge part of Medicare's expenditures is paid for hospital level care at the end of life, in patients who often too sick to benefit from such care. The fact that 63 percent of our elderly spend time in the hospital during their last month of life, and that such end-of-life splurging eats up a huge chunk of Medicare's budget without saving life or improving quality,[327][328] shows that this futile gasp of thorough care within the expensive hospital walls at the ends of someone's life makes no medical sense. Doctors and hospitals profit from such aggressive care, but the patient and the system are not quite as fortunate.

## Why is There so Much Hospitalization?

As we have discussed, studies show that a vast majority of elderly people prefer to die at home and not in a hospital, but very often their wishes are ignored as the teeth of America's aggressive medical mentality overtake patient preference.[329][330][331] There are many reasons that the hospital has become the destination of choice for those most ill, even those who have explicitly stated that they do not wish to be hospitalized. Some of the fault is more systemic, some is more patient-centric, but all of it is exacerbated by a Medicare system that encourages hospitalization through various means. Although CMS has initiated measures to curb hospital admissions, and although the dangers of hospitalization are well known to most of my patients and their families, Medicare's payment policies push people through the hospital's front door, sometimes against their will, sometimes as willing partners, even for conditions we know are treated more effectively and at a lower cost at home.

Fisher, who studies regional variation of care within the Medicare population, found that regions of the country with increased numbers of hospital beds and higher specialist concentrations are more likely to hospitalize the elderly. Such regional disparity is not impacted by diagnosis or the extent of illness. These high spending hospitals will cost Medicare more money per patient because they deliver more intensive care, care that much of the population would consider thorough. But as Fisher has shown, hospitals that spend the most money in the last six months of someone's life have a 2–6 percent increase in death rate compared to low-spending hospitals, irrespective of the degree of medical illness.[332]

But the perception of hospitals is quite different. Just last month a ninety-plus-year-old patient of mine presented to the office with increased confusion and weakness. I suggested to his son that he may have had a stroke, but that hospitalization would not be necessary, since there was nothing we could accomplish in a hospital that would alter his chance of recovery. Instead I suggested he move to a nursing home-rehab unit for a few weeks until he improved. The son agreed at first, but then was persuaded otherwise by those who know better (friends, family, the Internet) and he sent his dad to the hospital for a more thorough evaluation. In addition, although he did not verbalize it, the hospital would have cost him nothing, while a rehabilitation stay or home care could have cost him many thousands of dollars in out-of-pocket expenses not covered by Medicare. I pleaded with him to get his dad home, but he believed that his dad needed a good looking over before coming home. His dad never did come home. He died in the hospital, from complications created by the hospital, and not from his small stroke. His son did not blame the hospital, and in fact felt just the opposite: he told me that his dad must have been very sick to have died, and it was a good thing that he was in the hospital, which gave him the best chance of living. Such is a misconception that fills the hospital wards with so many elderly people who should not be there.

A few of my patients and their families buy into the notion that the hospital is the best place to go. I have patients who call 911 several times a month, are treated in the emergency room for minor complaints such as elevated blood pressure or dizziness and, several thousand dollars later, after exposure to significant risk, are sent home. Sometimes they are admitted when their story is good enough, and they are more than happy to see a half dozen specialists and have an ample helping of tests in the hope of fixing problems that have been plaguing them for months or years. Medicare pays for the hospital without asking questions. If my patients want to go there every day, Medicare puts up no barriers. And it is typically cheaper for them to sit in the hospital than to find transportation to see their doctor. Many of my patients and their families truly believe that hospital level of care gave them or their loved one the best chance of living. This is an idea so deeply imbedded into our zeitgeist that nothing I can ever say will dissuade them from their thinking. Few of them realize that, in too many cases, the hospital actually precipitated the very spiraling crisis that they are lauding the hospital for heroically and thoroughly ameliorating.

But too many of my patients, even the ones who with their families believe in minimalist palliative care, eventually often find themselves in the hospital despite expressing very firm wishes otherwise. Part of it is fear that, when serious illness pops its ugly head, hospitalization is necessary to avert death. Not knowing what else to do, they call 911. It occurs in a moment of panic, even among people who disdain hospital care. Other families do it out of necessity. They cannot afford to keep their loved one at home, cannot afford a rehabilitation stint, and so resort to the hospital as the one place where their loved one can get care and have that care paid by Medicare. Why is that? Hospitals provide twenty-four-hour care, paid for by Medicare A, while no part of Medicare pays for adequate care at home.

To obtain sufficient care out of the hospital, patients either have to pay for home health aides, something that Medicare will not reimburse, or spend time in the subacute unit of a nursing home, something for which Medicare A will pay **but only after a three-night stay in a hospital,** as we have discussed. Patients can obtain limited nursing services and rehabilitation at home through Medicare A, but not the custodial care they often need, not the IV fluids if they need that, and often not even the medicines. Not everyone has the financial and human resources to provide home care, especially when Medicare is barely helping, and when a far better reimbursed option exists within the hospital walls.

Ironically, not only is it safer for elderly patients with conditions like pneumonia to stay at home, but it is far less expensive to the health care system to provide such care at home, even if home care is more expensive for the patient himself. The cost of treating pneumonia is approximately $10 billion per year, most of which is spent on the elderly, and 92 percent of which is spent on hospital care.[333] In a study of hospital-level in home services, such as that provided by some VA sites, there was a substantial decrease in cost without decline in treatment quality for those treated at home not only for pneumonia but also for CHF, COPD, and cellulitis.[334] Thus home care would be feasible for the elderly if Medicare paid for it, and it would be both medically beneficial and cost saving. Instead, Medicare's payment system encourages just the opposite.

Medicare similarly nudges doctors like me to send my sick patients to the hospital rather than to arrange home services, because hospitalization is the easiest path for us to take. As Ira Byock observes: "Trying to manage the myriad problems of a chronically ill patient in a busy office can feel like juggling Jell-O on a busy city street corner in a rainstorm. The easiest, safest, and most efficient thing for a doctor to do is to send such acutely ill patients to the hospital."[335] We simply do not have time to jump over all the hurdles that Medicare has tossed across our path to help our patients stay at home. Arranging home health care is an onerous burden requiring calls and paperwork, and separate calls have to be made to agencies that provide home health aides, if they are even available. Medicines must be called in. Sometimes patients need equipment, such as oxygen or nebulizer machines, each of which requires more calls and paperwork. All this has become even more difficult under new Medicare and ACA rules. Usually these services cannot even start until the following day. I and my office staff have spent countless hours on many occasions trying to arrange services at home, often only to find that the patients cannot afford such services, or the services are not available, or the paperwork must be redone because a portion of it did not comply with regulations. Nothing in the Medicare universe helps us arrange home care; instead, it makes such an endeavor virtually impossible. Contrarily, if we tell our patients to call 911 and go to the hospital, our total cost in time is measured in minutes, and our patients feel that we are helping them. Many patients have thanked me for sending them to the hospital just in the nick of time to save their lives. For them and for me, hospitalization is the only feasible route available when they are fairly ill, even though I know that it is not the best route for my patients or for our health care system.

Hospitalization also incentivizes doctors in other ways. Hospital reimbursement is good for doctors, who are expected to see hospitalized patients every day; many of us can see more patients at a higher reimbursement in the hospital than in an office. For specialists and generalists alike, hospital medicine is lucrative. Now many hospitals are hiring their own doctors, presumably to keep some of that money within their own coffers. Hospital monetary arrangements are much too complicated for this book, and many hospitals are always proclaiming that they are on the precipice of financial collapse, but their doctors do quite well, as do their CEOs. An August 2013 article in the *Baltimore Sun* showed that most CEOs of Maryland hospitals earn well over $600,000, with thirteen of them earning over a million dollars a year.[336] Certainly, Medicare has been very kind to American hospitals.

## Moving in a Sensible Direction

Even as geriatric doctors know that hospital care must be curbed for the good of our patients' health and for the survival of Medicare, even as we hope for actual reform that will enable us to treat our patients safely in their homes, which is what so many of us and our patients prefer, we do realize that any assault on hospital care will be met with resistance. That is because hospitals perform a vital role in our society. An American Hospital Association website spells out the economic value of hospitals. They employ over 5.3 million people, are the second largest source of private sector jobs in the country, spend $320 billion on goods and services, and create over two trillion dollars of economic activity. That economic activity creates ripple effects that spur even more jobs and economic growth.[337] Hospitals also are the primary training arena for medical students and residents, are essential for medical research, and perform vital medical services that are both necessary and lifesaving.

Moving a large portion of geriatric care outside of the hospital walls will certainly cause these institutions economic injury, even though hospitals will still control a large sector of health care provision, from trauma care, to surgery, to obstetrics, to the acute care of heart attacks. But hospitals do not have to abandon geriatric care; they simply have to offer more sensible care. To some extent that is already occurring and, as we will show, some Medicare and ACA reforms are making small attempts to avert hospitalization among the frail elderly.

ACE (Acute Care for the Elders) units in some hospitals are already accomplishing that goal by providing quality geriatric care at lower cost and with improved outcomes. In an ACE unit, such as one described at Ohio State, older patients felt to be most at risk for functional decline are identified and treated by an interdisciplinary team expert in geriatric care. There are multiple such units sprouting all over the country.[338] ACE units have been shown to decrease functional decline, decrease the use of restraints, and increase the satisfaction of patients, caregivers, nurses, and doctors. There are also decreased falls, less delirium/confusion, and more likelihood of a patient being discharged home rather than to a nursing home. There is some evidence that ACE units can decrease length of stay and cost, although these findings are not consistent.[339] [340] Such units allow patients to be discharged from hospitals in better health than occurs in traditional hospital units and with less likelihood that they will be readmitted for the same diagnosis.[341]

Another movement in some hospitals is to establish geriatric emergency rooms that specifically meet the needs of older patients with moderate illness. Holy Cross Hospital in Maryland established the first such unit, and it is popular with both patients and providers of care. In the geriatric ER a team of geriatric doctors, nurse practitioners, nurses, and social workers try to address the more global needs of patients. The rooms are larger and designed for the needs of the elderly, with heated thick mattresses, easily accessed electronics, and increased space for family consultations.[342] A 2007 article describes how such emergency rooms can help meet the very complicated needs of older patients,[343] although no studies to date have demonstrated improved outcome or reduced cost from using geriatric emergency rooms. As with ACE units, the hope in a geriatric ER would be that a patient is given the specific treatment required to help her surmount an acute illness, such as IV fluids if she cannot eat, and then sent home with in-home care. As noted, though, even under the umbrella of its recent reform thrust, Medicare remains stingy with regard to home care, and for patients it is much less costly to receive services at a hospital than at home.

Perhaps the most promising innovation hospitals may consider in caring for the elderly would be the establishment of palliative care programs. The number of such programs has increased nationally. A study of eight hospitals with palliative care services showed that the cost of care was markedly reduced compared to traditional care.[344] Palliative hospital care represents an approach that emphasizes function, satisfaction, and comfort rather than the more aggressive and specialized treatment to which most elderly patients are subjected in hospitals.

One can envision geriatric ER's and ACE units with palliative care teams in which the ill elderly can be cared for compassionately to stabilize them before sending them home with home care services. Currently hospitals are potentially harmful destinations for older patients that offer no measurable medical benefit in many cases. Medicare both generously reimburses hospital care and encourages hospitalization through its payment system. Medicare does very little to help with home care and other focused medical interventions provided outside an aggressive hospital setting. The cost of hospital care for the elderly is one of the most potent factors that are draining Medicare of its funding without delivering any value. For that reality to change, Medicare must orchestrate a saner course.

# 5

# LONG-TERM CARE: THE UNWITTING GERIATRIC ICU

"Too often in these institutions, there is more attention
paid to disease than to persons, more scientific curiosity
about the machinery of the body than consideration
of the human values that make life worthwhile."
-Hadler, *Rethinking Aging*

Long-term care is the soul of geriatrics. It is in long-term care facilities that we care for the frailest of the elderly. We see them in their homes at all hours of the day, we joke with them, sit with them, and often hold their hands during every extreme of their emotions. Many of them are demented, and as they drift away from reality we become an integral part of their new lives, and those of their loved ones. I take care of people in many assisted living and nursing facilities. Some are small homes managed by good-natured owners and nursing aides, others are large national chains or independent facilities with administrators, nurses, and aides who are equally devoted to their residents. We all work as a team, and all of us enjoy immersing ourselves in the lives of those for whom we care. It is a huge responsibility, and one that none of us takes lightly. Nothing gives us more joy than having our patients smile when we walk by, or talk to us about their past lives, or walk with us serenely on the way to breakfast. I have become so close to all of the people in my facilities—social workers, aides, nurses, therapists, administrators, patients, families, and so many others—that when I walk in, typically early in the morning, I have a smile on my face; it is as if I am entering my own home. It engenders a feeling of comfort and warmth. Caring for the residents of long-term care is a passion that many of us in geriatrics share.

There are many shapes of long-term care. Assisted-living facilities typically house those who can perform some tasks on their own, although increasingly they are being occupied by people with significant mental and physical limitations. Many larger homes have separate dementia units, where more severely demented residents live in various arrangements. Assisted-living facilities vary in cost, typically being less expensive than nursing homes. They are less regulated than nursing homes; cannot care for skilled residents, as we will discuss; and typically are self-pay, rarely allowing more than a few residents for whom Medicaid will pay the bills. Nursing homes typically are much larger. Some have hundreds of beds, ventilation units, and even dialysis on the premises. Nursing homes are highly regulated and they hire an expansive staff to care for residents and to comply with regulations. The typical resident of a nursing home is more impaired, typically very demented and requiring a significant amount of custodial care. When residents exhaust their funds, Medicaid may pay for their stay, although many nursing homes actually lose money on their Medicaid residents. Where they earn more money is in Medicare payment, something that engenders yet another layer of regulation. Any Medicare patient who stays three nights in a hospital who then has a skilled need (nursing care or physical therapy) can qualify for up to one hundred days of services within a nursing home paid by Medicare. Very often nursing homes need a significant number of skilled Medicare residents to offset the cost of their unskilled Medicaid residents.

If there are any places on this earth where older patients should be treated with a minimalistic approach, where adverse outcomes should be expected and ameliorated palliatively without looking for cause or ascribing blame, where trips to the hospital should be avoided at all costs, where medicines and tests should be shunned, and where comfort and dignity should be the only goals, it is at long-term care facilities. And yet, it is at such facilities that I have seen aggressive care reach its zenith. We will primarily be discussing nursing homes in this chapter, since assisted-living facilities are less burdened by state regulations and by Medicare rules, but assisted-living facilities are not immune from the shackles placed on all long-term care facilities, and many of them too are forced to maintain a very aggressive stance.

Everything we know about geriatrics tells us that number chasing, overly thorough testing and treatment, and hospitalization in this population is counterproductive, often leading to more harm than good. And yet facility patients are flooded by thorough care incessantly, much more than they would be if they lived at home. Although hardly alone in its culpability, Medicare plays a large role in pushing long-term care patients on a path of aggression. The three-day hospital rule establishes a dichotomy of class within the nursing home world, whereby those patients who have had their tickets punched in the hospital are more profitable to a nursing home than those who have not. In all facilities it is far less expensive for facility and patient alike to hospitalize very ill residents, also due to Medicare's payment model.

Long-term care facilities are also burdened by extensive regulations that reward "thorough" care and hospitalization and rebuke a more palliative approach. This, more than even Medicare's rules, sews a zeitgeist of aggression into the culture of long-term care. As with Medicare's quality indicators we discussed in chapter 1, the regulatory environment utilizes numbers and scales to assess quality. Whether from state or federal regulations or Medicare's own regulatory assessment tools, these quality indicators span hundreds of pages and are difficult for even the most seasoned administrators to fully comprehend. But the upshot of their message is that poor outcomes are not tolerated, that every facet of an elderly resident's health must be constantly monitored and maintained in the "normal" range, and that failure to comply with the regulations can lead to very damaging consequences. In my experience, compliance with regulatory demands exhausts more time from front line staff than does patient care; charting has become the primary activity on a nursing home floor. Even more significantly, all of us who care for the residents have to worry more about numbers and regulatory deficiencies than about the health and well-being of our patients.

The modus operandi of long term care is specialization. Although specialist doctors do not typically meander the halls of long term care facilities, and the preponderance of patients there are treated by geriatric primary care doctors who are well versed in palliative care, long-term care culture is one of myopic intensity, where a holistic outlook dissolves amid a thorough assault on every ailment, numerical deviation, and complaint exhibited by the frail elderly residents and those who care for them. Palliative care exists only when patients are deemed to be on the verge of death and enrolled in hospice. As is common in specialized environments, patients are carved up into diagnoses and conditions, each one viewed independently from the others, and each one treated aggressively. Tests and procedures are common within the walls of long-term care, with lab and x-ray technicians making frequent trips there, medications tossed at patients for every numerical blip or complaint, and hospitalization being a natural consequence of medical problems that become difficult to control. Short of the hospital itself, long-term care facilities are the most specialized settings in which I have practiced.

Of course, from everything we have discussed in this book, one has to wonder why the specialized model of care has taken root in long-term care, when its frail elderly inhabitants are most potentially harmed by narrowly focused aggressive care, and when palliation would seem to be most humane and effective. For instance, is it truly necessary to check blood pressures and sugars, often several times a day, and to assure that those pressures fall within a preordained range lest the nurses become alarmed and demand immediate intense treatment? What evidence exists that such thorough numerical monitoring actually benefits the frail elderly and that its treatment helps quality of life or even longevity? And if an older patient passes out, appears more tired, presents with stroke-like symptoms, or becomes more confused, what evidence exists that exposing such elderly patients to copious testing and hospitalization, where precise causes of each problem are ascertained by probing their aged bodies, will improve outcome and quality? And yet, that is what happens regularly in long-term care. We react to every deviation from the norm, and we toss the gamut of specialized care at them, usually without regard to outcome, and always without regard to how such treatment will impact the patient as a whole. All of this is done in a stressed and emotionally charged atmosphere that only exacerbates a patient's decline and a family's suffering. And Medicare pays for it all. While some Medicare reform is targeting the excessive hospitalization to which long-term care residents are subjected, nothing has been suggested to alter the specialized model of care within such facilities and to change the rules and financial realities that promote such aggressive care.

Ironically, those who manage the long-term care facilities in which I work, from owners to administrators, from nurses to aides, from social workers to nurse practitioners and doctors, do not endorse the aggressive cloud under which we have been asked to work. Some of the most progressive, creative, and humane geriatric thinkers I have ever encountered are the owners and directors of long-term care facilities, one of whom helped me to start my practice and who has guided me along the way, inspiring me with his conception of an ideal geriatric universe that he has tried so hard to implement against a resistive tide. We are all victims of a system that has morphed into something other than what it was designed to be. There is little we can do to change that reality. I belong to a wonderful organization called the American Medical Director's Association (AMDA), and have learned a great deal under its tutelage. The doctors in AMDA are devoted to making long-term care more patient oriented and sensible. They get it, and try very hard to enact meaningful reform. But even they are small fish in the politicized and emotional environment of

Medicare reimbursement and regulation, where reason often falls prey to an entrenched belief that with sufficient regulation, and with number chasing and problem fixing, we can transform the residents of long-term care from frail people at the end of their lives to vibrant souls who are perpetually well. Unfortunately, such arrogant thinking has had the opposite effect, at great cost to patients and society alike.

## Regulation

There is always a healthy debate in this country about how much regulation is too much. In the nursing home world, that answer is obvious to many of us who practice geriatrics: the **quantity** of regulations in nursing homes, and to a lesser extent assisted-living facilities, is excessive, and the **quality** of such regulation is both poor and counterproductive. Nursing homes are some of the most highly regulated institutions in the country.[345] In fact, regulations frequently trump the good patient care that nursing homes are trying to promote. Facilities spend excessive money and resources to make sure they are in compliance with the hundreds of regulations, so they have much less money and resources to spend to take care of their residents, such as to hire more aides and to assure their retention.

What are the regulations? Before my first state survey as a medical director I saw the facility director and several nurses walking around with a tape measure to determine if the spacing of items on the wall was within the guidelines. Even though the nursing home was contending with its usual array of significant clinical problems among its residents, the surveyors that year were focusing on measurements, and thus the facility had to devote more resources to that meaningless issue.

Every fall; every piece of tissue paper skin that tears in a ninety-year-old; every resident who requires a sedative to keep him from screaming all night; every piece of paper that is not signed in the right place at the right time; every chart sitting on the wrong part of a desk; not enough pain medicine; too much pain medicine; constipation from pain medicine; every mistake that occurs, however inadvertent and minor; every complaint by an angry family member; all of these cause consternation among nursing home administrators because any one of them can lead to a regulatory error, which can trigger a large fine, which can downgrade a facility in its rating, and which can precipitate financial hurt. I am contacted throughout the day and night by many facilities, often with very minor issues like a weight change, a slightly elevated blood pressure, a normal lab result, or a fall; I am asked to respond and provide a plan of care. These calls or emails can exceed the number of patients I care for in a home on any given day. Virtually all of them can wait until we come to the home in the next day or two, but regulatory exigency pushes reluctant nurses to let us know about them immediately, and we must respond with a plan of correction that can be documented and charted, all in the name of regulatory compliance.

I conducted an exhaustive literature search to determine if any evidence exists tying nursing home regulation to quality. Unfortunately, the answer to that query is predicated on how quality is defined. Since regulations define quality by numbers—how many falls, how many psychiatric medicines people are on, how many urine infections, how many forms are not signed—then clearly quality by that definition is improved with the regulations. It is a self-fulfilling conclusion, and one that seems to have hampered the true objectivity of any study that assesses the quality of care in long-term care facilities. But do those numbers truly represent quality? To me, more significant measures of patient quality— happiness, social interaction, energy, fewer outbursts by residents, fewer trips to the hospital, less pain—are not genuinely addressed. Several studies that do take a broader view of geriatric care note a disappointing relationship between quality of care and the regulatory environment.[346] [347] To me, using the commonsense measures we have addressed in this book as indicators of quality geriatric care, regulation not only does not contribute to better care, it actually detracts from it.

There is also a second layer of regulation that exhausts resources within a nursing home. To be paid by Medicare for skilled services, and to achieve the highest payment that Medicare allows, facilities must comply with a complex set of rules, many of which also require copious documentation of time, numbers, scales, and grades. As with state regulatory rules, the failure of a nursing home to comply with Medicare rules can be financially perilous. Thus homes hire a squadron of staff to help as much with regulation compliance as with patient care. Any visit to a nursing home, or even assisted-living, nursing station will typically find doctors and nurses sitting in front of computers charting and compiling data even more than actively caring for our patients. While we enjoy each other's company as we sit for hours mindlessly entering information into preset templates, we would rather be sitting with our patients or having more time to talk to families. Regulations, however, make that impossible.

## Number Obsession

Numbers in particular are placed under a microscope in facilities. They are easy to measure, and thus easy to regulate, even if they typically are bereft of any clinical significance. Today I was told that an assisted-living patient was on the regulatory radar because, according to a county social worker who was scrutinizing the facility, his blood pressure was too high and he should have a diagnosis of hypertension and be on blood pressure medicine. In my opinion the pressure was perfectly fine and we had no reason to treat it, let alone to even check it. What the regulator was requesting would have been detrimental to the patient, for reasons we have already discussed. The social worker went ever further, arguing that since the patient had a diagnosis of high cholesterol on her problem list, we were being negligent in not having her on statin drugs and checking her cholesterol labs tests periodically. We satisfied the regulator by removing both diagnoses from the problem list and by my writing a note explaining that the pressure and cholesterol were normal for her age and medical condition.

I have many constructive debates with nurses about numbers; often I am hounded by various voices in a facility because I refuse to treat what they consider high sugars and high blood pressure. I beg the nurses to stop checking blood pressure so often and I try hard to prevent any but the most essential sugar checks. I cite studies, which we have discussed in this book, demonstrating that aggressive treatment of hypertension and diabetes in frail elderly residents of long-term care facilities leads to worse functional outcomes, but those facts do not deflect the reality of long-term care regulations, even though the nurses and I are almost always in agreement. When a regulator spots "untreated" high blood pressure or diabetes, or vital signs and labs tests that are not being ordered in sufficient quantity, then she may fault a facility and instigate a painful and potential expensive citation process. When regulators play doctor and set the rules, then nurses really have no choice but to comply.

Anything less than an urgent approach to numerical abnormality is called "delayed response" and could lead to regulatory consequences. The same panicked posturing is expected for every change in condition among long-term care residents. Thus, even for a cold, nursing home residents may get x-rays and antibiotics and immediate calls into doctors. For constipation I have been called past midnight, because the nurse is concerned that a few more hours without a bowel movement will be considered a delayed response. Cuts that can be treated with a bandage are urgent. Falls, headaches, confusion, pain, congestion, diarrhea, or someone just not feeling well: all are common in older people, especially the frail ones who reside in long-term care, but all are considered urgent issues that require immediate notification and treatment. Such thorough posturing unwittingly manufactures a culture of aggressive care in virtually every realm of long-term care medicine.

## Weight Loss and the Overseers of Regulation

Weight is another number tracked closely by facilities because deviations from "normal" are judged harshly by the regulatory process. Although weight loss is common with aging, especially in demented patients, in the facility world it is unacceptable. So we check weights incessantly. When the weight drops, we draw labs. We flood patients with supplements. We add medicines that may help increase appetite. We may order tests or even consult specialists. We talk to the family about shoving a feeding tube into their loved one's gut lest they die of starvation. We geriatric doctors know that such an aggressive assault on a frail body will help neither longevity nor quality of life, and the fact is that feeding tubes actually do not save lives but harm them.[348] [349] [350] But that does not stop regulators from demanding an explanation about why old demented residents are losing weight, while insisting that something be done to curb that inevitable weight loss. Rather than focus on comfort and dignity and offering their residents peace in their final years, facilities are pushed by regulators to insist on a thorough approach to an inevitable problem of aging.

At one nursing home where I worked, a ninety-plus-year-old severely demented patient stopped eating. Even with help she was not interested in eating anything. Different appetite stimulants were given, tests were done, and assessments were made to assure she was not constipated or in pain. She was very happy and interactive, just not hungry. So she lost weight, something that the regulators do not like to see. The family all understood her level of dementia. They wanted her kept comfortable, maybe even put on hospice, so they asked us to stop weighing her and forcing her to eat. But then a social worker found a copy of her living will, written twenty years earlier, stating that she would want artificial food if she stopped eating. She had never altered that document. So the administrator and medical director became involved, and they stated that this happy, demented person in her nineties would need a feeding tube to get nutrition. They threatened to bring the family to court, mostly to protect themselves from regulations that forced them to act as such. The family was livid, knowing that the patient would not want such aggressive care, and neither did they. Eventually we procrastinated and fabricated excuses until the patient peacefully died. This frequent scenario smacks the face of common sense and good geriatric care. But it is what our nursing homes have become.

I remember another tube feed incident where the facility itself almost pushed a patient and her son to do what they knew was contrary to their wishes and to common sense. I had been taking care of an elderly woman for several years, and she had a severe swallowing disorder causing her to spend nearly two hours to finish even a simple meal. She was willing to live with that problem and actually coped quite well, neither losing weight nor choking on her food. Her son, a great guy, fully supported her. One day, though, she became ill with a respiratory infection and decompensated. She could not swallow at all. She finally agreed to surgery to fix her swallowing problem. The surgery was set up for three weeks, and her son and I agreed that for that time she would be safer in our nursing home facility where she could receive more care. But then an unanticipated assault ensued.

First the nurses were concerned by how slowly and painfully she was eating, something in fact that had not changed much from her baseline. But due to increased surveillance they witnessed every painful swallow, every bout of regurgitation. They hovered over her and fueled her anxiety, which only exacerbated her swallowing issues. They weighed her and found that she was too thin. They called me, questioning if she was safe to swallow at all, if she needed more medicines, if she should be denied food completely, if she should have a feeding tube placed. Her blood pressure increased every day, and she became more confused and agitated. A speech therapist was consulted, who similarly questioned her safety. That caused nurses to check her even more, marching into her room day and night with visages of angst and beeping blood pressure cuffs rolling by their sides. They called me and her son with panic and regularity, telling us that she was choking, that she was coughing, reading her blood pressures and weights, and requesting medicines, x-rays, even hospitalization. Her son became more anxious.

"Maybe we need to get her to a hospital," he asked me one day. "Maybe they're right."

"Just hold the course," I told him. "Nothing has changed. She is fine."

Then came the director of nursing and social workers, asking her if she wanted a feeding tube, telling her that she may die without it. Her anxiety level accentuated even further. The calls to us increased. Then the medical director intervened. A doctor himself, whose role in long-term care was to assure that all doctors complied with state and facility regulations, and to assure that facility physicians adhered to quality geriatric care (two goals that often are contradictory), he directly inserted himself into the situation. He talked to the patient and son and told them that she may well die if she did not get a tube put in her stomach to feed her immediately, that waiting for the surgery could be fatal, and that he could arrange for the tube to be put in. Certainly he was acting at the request of the administrators, who feared reprisals from regulators, and who were uncomfortable with a woman who could have an adverse outcome. Of course, the son became frantic, and the level of anxiety literally exploded.

I told the son not to worry. I came in early the next morning and wrote a two-page note in the chart explaining that the medical director was completely out of line to insert himself in a situation he did not understand, that the nurses and administrators needed to back off, and that the patient was doing fine by every objective criteria we had, including weight (which had not dropped since admission) and blood work. My words were sharp, and I was reprimanded by the medical director and in fact was almost fired for my actions. Two weeks later the woman had her surgery, she went home with twenty-four-hour care rather than return to the nursing home, and she lived very well (out of hospitals and subsequent nursing homes) for the rest of her life that spanned many years.

## Falls: The Benefits of Front-Line Staff

Many residents move to long-term care because they fall, and thus it is not a surprise that they are still falling after they arrive. Many have dementia and try to get up even though they should not. They need to go to the bathroom and will not or cannot wait. Sometimes their blood pressure is too low, they are on too many medicines, or they are on medicines known to cause falls.[351] [352] [353] Having more nursing aides around, and having residents in activities that are monitored, can mitigate the chance of falling. But there are never enough aides to help everyone, and regulatory law prevents restraining residents. Even when medicines are used to calm them, that only increases their rates of falls. And because falls trigger regulatory alarms, facilities have to be very attentive to them. Fall prevention programs can help,[354] but their implementation requires money and trained personnel, something lacking in facilities that have to devote so many resources to nonclinical activities, such as regulatory and Medicare compliance.

I was amazed one day while at a nursing home to learn how its corporate administration was looking into the reason that so many nursing home residents were falling. Too many falls is problematic on many levels, but in terms of the financial bottom line falls can lead to deficiencies on surveys that can lead to a downgrading of a facility's rating that can lead to a drop in census and less money. So when the parent company of the nursing home decided to spend $500,000 to hire a consultant to ascertain the cause of falls, I was floored. I remember sitting around with some of the nursing aides one morning talking about it.

"They fall," one of them said, "because they all have to go to the bathroom at the same time, and we can't all be there at that time for every one of them." She had been at the nursing home for a long time, one of the few aides who actually stayed for more than a year. "I know I have to see Mrs. S. right away when she gets up, then hurry to Mr. W., then I told Mrs. L. to be patient, and I know she usually won't try to get up until I get there while the other two will, but sometimes she just does anyway."

"If they took that money they're paying that consultant and just hired some more aides," another one said, "then the problem would be solved tomorrow."

"If they took some of that money and paid us just a little more, then we would stick around and that would solve the problem too," another chimed in.

Yes, the nursing aides solved the whole problem in a matter of minutes. Pay nurses and aides enough to induce them to remain loyal so that they stay, thereby assuring that they know their patients and that their patient/families know them. Make sure there are enough nurses and aides so that they can help people when help is needed, and that they get a break once in a while, because taking care of an old nursing home resident who slaps you and who greets you with a diaper full of excrement is not the most pleasant way to spend a day, and there are always a few of those in every nursing home with whom aides have to contend. And treat the nurses and aides with dignity and respect; too often aides are blamed when problems occur, they are fired, they are reprimanded, and the system chews them up like they are just pegs in some grand board game.

The cost of having more and happier front-line staff is minimal compared to what some facilities pay their executives and consultants to try to solve weighty issues such as fall prevention, and that cost translates into a better facility. When the average annual turnover of nursing aides is over 85 percent, quality will clearly decline.[355] [356] There is nothing more revealing than the reaction of patients and families when they lose their trusted aide. In my experience patients demonstrate sadness, consternation, fear, and usually a worsening of behavior. Regulators do not measure that level of quality, but we see it every day.

Interestingly, while good aides clearly help improve a facility and resident/family satisfaction, that does not necessarily translate to a better regulatory outcome. One study I read suggested that increasing the number of nursing aides in a facility does not lead to fewer deficiencies on a state survey[357] likely because the survey process is measuring parameters that do not reflect the quality that aides deliver. Aides can engage with residents in interesting and personalized activities, walk with them, sing and laugh with them, make them feel happy and autonomous, and be more attuned to their needs, but there may be no appreciable improvement in most survey quality indicators. In fact, when facilities permit residents to have more freedom, where they are not watched like hawks and they are involved in creative dementia programs, falls may increase, especially when there are not enough aides to personally watch every high-risk resident all the time.

## Medicines and Regulatory Schizophrenia

Pharmaceutical regulations are also very vexing and cost facilities money and time to assure compliance. These regulations are often contradictory, demanding more lab tests, number measurements, and medicines, even as they chastise polypharmacy. Patients are not permitted to be in pain, and yet the regulations required to maintain patients on pain medicines are arduous and time-consuming for everyone in the facilities. Similarly, facilities would like to assure that very confused, agitated, and even delusional residents are relatively calm, do not bother other residents, do not fall, and shower and eat regularly, but facilities are often denied the tools to make that happen. Nurses and nursing aides are put in a horrible position as some residents lash out at them or start to run off, and it requires half of a floor of staff to try redirect them without using restraints or coercion, which the regulations forbid. They also do not typically have enough time to provide the personal attention to calm and redirect confused residents. So we treat them with medicines, most of which are not indicated for dementia, carry a black box warning, and lead to sedation and falls. Regulations frown on such medicines, while at the same time frowning on what would happen should those medicines not be given. It's damned if you do and damned if you don't in the medical universe of long-term care.

Every medicine carries a potential risk, and every medicine can lead to regulatory issues if specified rules about its use are not followed. Some medicines require lab surveillance, some require attempts at stopping them periodically, some need special forms that doctors must complete frequently, others are felt to be inappropriate for the elderly and require us to justify their use. Therefore facilities have to employ specific long-term care pharmacies to dispense their medicines and provide a consultant pharmacist. The pharmacist reviews charts regularly and instructs facilities on how to follow the regulatory rules. While a little input from a pharmacist is always invited, and the pharmacists with whom I work are wonderful people who educate us and help us to remain compliant, these guidelines, which flow to us frequently in the form of reports we have to address, are born of regulatory needs, not of any true adherence to quality geriatric care. They also cost patients more money, since medicine prices are escalated to cover the regulatory expense, and they cost the facility both time and money. They also lead to excessive number obsession, test ordering, and second guessing.

Facilities are also forbidden from dispensing over-the-counter medicines without a doctor's order. If my knee hurts I can take a Tylenol, and if my nose runs I can take a Claritin. But long-term care residents require doctor orders for everything, even a vitamin. If we add a bunch of basic over-the-counter medicines to the patient's list that can be dispensed as needed, that also causes consternation since facilities are judged too on how long their average resident's medicine list is. They must remain on four blood pressure medicines and a statin because we of course need to keep the numbers looking good, but God forbid we add a few medicines for constipation, pain, heartburn, or gas that they can get when they ask. Comfort takes a back seat to regulatory requirements and number fixing.

## The Survey: Regulation's Annual Alamo

In some distant past life I am sure that facility regulations were developed to prevent gross negligence and excess. Some facilities were certainly mistreating residents and were scamming the system. But these days, the vast majority of the facilities are doing their best to take care of a very sick patient population in a responsible and dignified way. I have never been to a facility that deserved anything but a very high passing grade on a state survey. All the nit-picking and inane regulations that are enforced by regulators are not designed to help facilities best care for their patients. Those regulations are built to satisfy regulatory requirements, which give birth not to improved quality but rather to increased costs and a compromised quality of care. While regulators can assess facilities at any time, and people are monitoring falls and dozens of other numbers regularly, the big survey occurs only once a year (and less frequently in assisted-living facilities). Survey day is never announced, but facilities are given a window of several months in which a squadron of regulators could potentially arrive, and there is always talk among the many facilities in a community speculating when the regulators may be nearby. Anxiety grips facilities as soon as a hint arrives that the regulatory team may be close. Nurses, social workers, and administrators spend long days and often some nights digging through charts, putting everything in its place, making sure that every bad outcome is accounted for and every paper is signed.

On survey day the entire facility essentially bows down to the all-powerful regulators, holding its collective breath as a small squadron enters the building, skewers the charts, talks to people, digs into every nook and cranny of the floor, and then starts handing out deficiencies. On our last survey, the regulators determined that some pages in a chart were not signed. A deficiency was allocated. The facility then spent the next few months not only fixing that problem, but developing a new system to assure that the problem did not occur again, and then proving to the regulators that the new system (a binder in which unsigned pages were kept for every doctor) was being used by sending them a plan of correction. It was a huge waste of money and time for nothing! And that was a good survey!

Last summer I spent days grappling with a survey result that cited us because our office note indicated that a patient was on an over-the-counter medicine but the facility chart did not have that medicine listed. This required hours of phone time, written letters, and meetings before it was resolved, although a deficiency was still handed to the facility. Recently I witnessed a survey team citing a facility because a two-hundred- pound woman fell on a nursing aide as the aide was trying desperately to transfer her out of the bed; the facility fired the aide, likely so blame could be deflected from it to her. On one occasion a daughter complained that her mom fell too many times. In reality, despite the aide's best efforts, the mom would try to get up as soon as the aide left the room. The regulators paid a visit. That aide was fired. On another occasion a facility received a survey deficiency because an aide was yelling loudly at a demented resident, even though the resident in question was deaf and refused to wear her hearing aids.

As soon as an annual survey is complete, the facility is already preparing for the next one. Facilities are given one to five stars based primarily on survey results. People like to put their loved ones in five-star facilities. So the facility administrator will do everything in his or her power to get to four or five stars. In addition to causing star reduction, survey deficiencies incur fines, some of which are very large. Deficiencies also mandate facilities to engage in a process that proceeds for several months after the survey, whereby they have to write a comprehensive evaluation of why they were deficient and what plan of correction they intend to implement to assure it does not happen again. I remember sitting in monthly quality assurance meetings as the charge nurse had to read her plan of correction month after month, explaining what was being done to fix the cited problem: having a cookie warming machine to give residents cookes in a patient care area, something the survey thought could be dangerous. Such deficiencies squander valuable time for nurses and aides who would rather concentrate on patient needs and talk about creative ways to care for their residents rather than having to focus on the placement of unplugged cookie warming machines.

Within the regulatory cloud we maintain our primary goal to help our patients. The nurses, social workers, and aides with whom I am lucky enough to work are passionate about patient care. They adore their residents, and truly understand how to care for them in the best possible way. It is to them who both I and patients' family members look for guidance and answers. In the best facilities where I work, they will comply with the regulations, but their hearts and minds lay elsewhere.

A few months ago I was giving a talk to nurses and aides about how to address demented residents who refuse care, are agitated, and are unable to be redirected. We discussed the need to avoid confronting demented residents when they resist certain aspects of care and not to stress them by arguing with them. We talked about psychiatric medicines, their side effects, and how regulations impact their use. And we talked about checking certain labs and tests and urines when residents do become more confused. One aide who had been there for a while told us how she dealt with one of the most agitated residents on the floor. The resident would not eat, and would not shower; she swung at people who tried to direct her. So the aide, who knew the resident and family well, learned something about her life. Before every shower day she told the resident that it was prom night, and that her prom date would be here soon. The resident lit up with glee, and cheerfully took a shower and dressed herself. Then she ate. This happened day after day. She did not need medicines, labs, tests, probes, blood pressure cuffs, consultants, or hospital admission to solve a very difficult problem. Rather, because she knew the resident well, because she asked the right questions, and because she cared, the underpaid nursing aide employed compassion and common sense to make someone very happy in her last months or years on this earth. It is very likely that the survey process would frown on her approach; after all, she did lie to the resident almost every day. But what the survey fails to grasp is that the best form of medicine is not a series of numbers and deficiencies that can be measured and charted, but rather it is something much more ephemeral. It is good geriatric care. It is love. And that comes very cheap.

## Expectations Gone Wild

In the nursing home environment, although most of my patients and their children truly value comfort and dignity as the primary goals of care, many others are imbued with a belief that number chasing and aggressive treatment are both appropriate and beneficial. I remember taking one of my older patients off a statin cholesterol drug when she developed a severe bronchitis and had trouble walking. This was a patient who requested frequent labs tests and medicines, and nothing I could say would dissuade her from the perception that more is better. But now, in the midst of her lung infection, I believed that the statin was actually causing her harm, so I persuaded her to stop it.

"That medicine could make you hurt more," I told her. "I'm going to remove it."

She acceded but was very sick, and I am not sure she fully comprehended the ramifications of my words.

Months later, having forgotten our conversation, a nurse told her that her statin was gone from her medicine list. She screamed at me, telling me that I was trying to kill her, that I didn't have any sense or knowledge, accusing me of not giving old people good care. I tried to explain that we could start it again, that being off a cholesterol medicine for a few months would cause no harm, and that at the time she benefited from its discontinuation. But she wanted none of my rationalizations; after all, someone had put her on that pill to save her life, and now I callously removed it. She immediately fired me and found a new doctor, one who was more thorough. I remember sitting at the nursing station a few weeks later, when she rolled in with her electric wheelchair. Pointing at me, but talking to the nurse, she said, "Does that nincompoop still work here?"

Several times a year I publish a newsletter in my practice discussing updated issues in geriatric care. This year I wrote my back page article on excessive care in the nursing home. Discussing recent studies and citing my own experience, I concluded that people in long-term care are better served through a palliative approach that does not emphasize fixing numbers and sending people to the hospital.

Soon enough I heard concerns voiced about my article. One of my patients asked another doctor if I was trying to kill people who got old, like Dr. Kevorkian. Another patient of mine brought over a written statement to me declaring that she wanted everything done for her should she get sick, so fearful was she that I would pull the plug the moment illness struck her. To these and other patients, the very notion that palliation could actually be beneficial falls in the face of every notion of good care in which they believe. My audacity in arguing for a minimalistic approach was interpreted as cruel and unfeeling.

The idea of long-term care as being a "rest home" or "convalescent home" has morphed over the decades. Now there can be no rest when monitors, needles, x-rays, and medicines are thrust at long-term care residents steadily. "Rest home" is the very antithesis of what these places have become.

Mrs. H. learned that lesson quickly. Her husband Mr. H.'s dementia progressed slowly. Mrs. H. kept him busy playing tennis, engaged with friends, and reading history books. But as his disease advanced, she watched his brilliant and energetic mind wilt away, and she saw her own vibrant life torn apart by his accelerating confusion and disability. During the early stages of his disease Mrs. H., who attended most of his appointments, made sure that her husband spent at least part of every visit with me alone. He always joked that the most annoying part of his disease was that the uneducated ladies with whom he ate dinner could talk and reason better than he could, even though they talked out of their asses. One day he told me point blank that if his Alzheimer's advanced to the point that his wife needed to care for him at the expense of her own life, or that he could not hold his own in a conversation, he intended to take out one of his guns and blow out his brains. His visage exuded absolute determination.

When I relayed his sentiments to his wife, she smiled and shrugged her shoulders. "Who can blame him?" she said to me.

Like so many spouses of my demented patients, Mrs. H. made a heroic stand against her husband's disease. She read about dementia, talked to me regularly about how to handle certain behavioral problems he exhibited, and kept her husband busy, always respecting his dignity. But unlike so many spouses, Mrs. H. knew when to say when. She did not chase elusive cures or flood him with feckless medicines. When their existence was transformed into a perpetual day-care center, when he embarrassed himself by soiling his pants in public or babbling nonsensically during conversations, Mrs. H. reluctantly moved the proud but bewildered man into a nursing home. She had cared for him for almost a decade at home, and now her husband barely could string together a meaningful sentence. He had moved well beyond the ability to kill himself or even generate such a complex thought. Mrs. H. asked me to stop all of his medicines and treat him for nothing but pain. She wanted to give him peace.

The nurses questioned her harsh stance; Mr. H. looked good, seemed happy, and was very engaging. But she knew he did not want to live this way. When he stopped eating, she told me that was his choice, and she wanted no intervention. When he developed pneumonia, she told me to keep him comfortable, not to give him antibiotics. People in the nursing home questioned her stance. From nurses to administrators, the nursing home pounced on her for neglecting her husband.

"They keep telling me I am doing the wrong thing," she told me, referring to the nursing home staff and administrators. "They tell me that I am letting him die."

We talked about it. She felt horribly guilty. Very often in my experience, even when a patient's family member reaches a decision to allow nature take its course, she is pushed hard to be more aggressive not only by the facility, but also by other family and friends. Mrs. H. was a very strong woman who held her own ground. She knew what was best for her husband, and when he did die he did so peacefully. Dementia is a tragic disease. Mrs. H. had lost her husband years earlier, but she could not mourn him. She stood by helplessly as her husband's illness ripped out his soul and left an empty hide in his place. This is the last thing he would have wanted. Finally, knowing that their love needed a release, she became a hero and let her husband go. But that approach did not sit well in the do-everything world of long-term care. In fact, to many it seemed cruel, as I heard in the echoes of the nursing home staff's chatter that followed his death, none of which was complementary to Mrs. H.

I recall another patient with severe dementia, Mrs. L., whose husband cared for her as best he could. Both were lovely people. But then when a sudden illness overcame and weakened her, he sent her to the nursing home. She did not recover. He made the conscious decision to treat her only for pain and discomfort, eschewing more aggressive care. His daughters were not happy with the decision. They talked to the nurses and learned that their mom had stopped eating and refused to walk. The nurses and staff outlined many steps that could be taken: blood tests, urine tests, chest x-rays, hospitalization. They told the daughters that their father refused all such care. One of the daughters talked to me and, with the permission of Mrs. L.'s husband, who was also my patient, I told them that I agreed with his decisions, as both he and his wife had told me that they did not want any extraordinary care once they had reached the end of life.

"How do you know she is at the end of life?" The daughter asked me. "How does he know? Why not give her a chance?"

I tried to explain to her that even if we found something wrong and we fixed it, there was a slim chance that her deteriorating body could be revived. We might delay her death, but it would not be for long. When an older person with dementia turns off, when she stops eating and interacting, we can mine for problems and repair them, one after another, but only at the cost of causing her pain and triggering even more problems, and never with the likelihood of inducing any real healing. She listened, but I do not think she accepted my words. The nurses told her that there were other options to explore. Her friends implored her to do more. How could her dad let mom die without a fight?

So she fought her dad, making him more miserable. He was very firm in his conviction, repeating to me and to his daughters that his wife had insisted that she not be treated with anything more than comfort should she become incapacitated. He had documents to prove it, which was very good because otherwise his stand would have been more difficult. So his daughter stopped talking to him. She also stopped talking to her sister, who decided to support her dad. When my patient finally died several weeks later, it took many months before the once very close family came back together.

I have seen countless families torn apart by such wrenching decisions. Many families of long-term care residents find it very difficult to abandon hope, which is how they perceive the relinquishing of an aggressive mentality, even if their loved one had previously told them to act otherwise. There is always more that can be done, more tests and treatments, even a hospital stay, that perhaps can reverse the slide that aging has instigated. They have heard stories about other people in similar circumstances who, when at death's door, were treated and cured. Society bombards them with tales of hope as long as they never abandon their fight. The nursing home environment only reinforces that mentality and eggs them on.

## Pushed to the Brink

It is almost twilight-zone-like for a geriatric doctor to watch all the medical attention being heaved upon the frailest residents of long-term care who are trying so hard to just be comfortable while probes and needles are being shoved into them, or the ambulance squad is throwing them on a gurney for a long, bumpy ride to the hospital. And that level of intensity pushes everyone—families, nurses, doctors, patients—into a state of mind whereby anxiety and high expectations completely obscure common sense and geriatric reality.

Because of regulatory rules, families often are bombarded by concerns about their loved ones from nurses and staff, especially if their family member has become more ill, and these families then start to worry. Sometimes they watch mom decline and wonder why, thinking there is more that could and should be done, that no one should ever die or decline without more of an effort, perhaps even a stay in the hospital. The long-term care environment feeds their angst. Once panic states to overtake reason, once the fable of hope supplants the reality of aging, then there is no turning back. As a doctor in those situations I am often barraged by emails and calls, from nurses, from families, even from other physicians. They crescendo in intensity, day and night, dramatizing the extent of the resident's medical collapse, requesting that more be done, often pushing for hospitalization. In my more idealistic youth I would try to convince them that staying put was the best approach, and sometimes I would come into the facility to try to be more persuasive. That approach could delay the inevitable for hours, maybe a day, but I soon learned that once the train of fear and panic takes over, it will never be stopped. Now I typically just give up and send them off to the hospital.

Just yesterday a ninety-three-year-old woman presented to the office with what seemed to be a small stroke, and I discussed the options of both hospitalization and nonskilled nursing home placement with her and her son. She adamantly opposed the hospital, but it took some convincing to persuade her son, who had heard that a patient must be sent to the hospital without pause if they had signs of stroke. Calling 911 would have been easy and my day would have been done. Instead we set up a CT scan that evening and arranged an admission to a long-term care facility, something that took hours of time, and something for which the family would have to pay. The next day a physical therapist told the son that not going to the hospital was a poor decision. He started to see a decline in his mom, something reinforced reluctantly by nursing. Vitals signs were abnormal. She could not swallow correctly. She likely became more nervous as everyone around her worried. A wave of anxiety consumed the son and the entire floor. Why wasn't she sent to the hospital? Were we just going to let her die? Somehow, as often happens, the hospital took on a magical power, as though when a ninety-three-year-old stroke victim rolls through its doors her ailments will be expunged miraculously. All our time and effort trying to treat this very elderly woman in the most palliative and humane way possible, and in total concert with her own wishes, collapsed in a matter of hours; an innuendo of doubt sparked the fire, and then more fuel intensified the flames, because in the world of long-term care there is always an abundance of kindling and very little available to extinguish a fire once it starts. She was whisked away to the hospital, and there was nothing we could do; in fact, if she survived three nights there, her ticket would be punched and the entire subacute stay would be financed by Medicare. As a colleague told me, it is senseless trying to stop it; I should have just called 911 yesterday.

With so many people magnifying every medical problem into a crisis, with so many people of authority evoking the specter of aggressive care, with so many rules and incentives shoving nursing home residents to the nearest hospital, with so much monitoring being done, with so low a level of tolerance for any clinical deterioration, with so many people hired not to care for patients but rather to watch over the regulatory landscape, and with so many families who start having unrealistic expectations, no wonder that thorough care becomes the norm. No wonder that ambulances and x-ray machines and lab technicians make incessant visits to the nursing home. No wonder that the level of anxiety and anger is always high, reflecting a shared frustration. And no wonder that the cost of geriatric care, both financially and personally, is so much steeper than anywhere else in the medical community.

What makes the facility atmosphere even worse is family frustration with long-term care. Many families I know who send their loved ones into assisted-living facilities or nursing homes do so reluctantly, often with their loved ones kicking and screaming and tossing blame at them. Clearly when they do make the decision for long-term care placement, families are driven by necessity; their parents can no longer safely or affordably live at home. Not everyone is so blessed as to have the Taunton Portuguese community, that can keep people like Mrs. A. at home, or the resources to hire round-the-clock help. And families have to pay huge fees to send their loved ones into long-term care facilities, something that often is very stressful as well. When finally the decision is made, and mom or dad is deposited in a small room with a roommate, most family members are already fried. They are struggling enough with their loved one's decline, and now are even more distraught that their loved one has to live the rest of her life in a small room with no autonomy, in a place many of them vowed never to be.

The anger and angst typically accelerate early in their loved one's stay. They come in to find mom sitting in a pool of urine. They learn she fell twice, that she did not eat her breakfast, that she slapped an aide. They see that a food tray is left by her side untouched and assume that no one attempted to feed her. They see that she sits in a chair staring at the wall much of the day. They witness other confused residents wandering into her room. They start to complain to the nurses, to spend more time there. They have lost so much control that they feel helpless and even guiltier. They start to question every aspect of mom's care.

All of this is augmented as they receive bills from the facility for hidden fees and exorbitant medication costs. They wonder how they will be able to afford this. Then they get calls requesting more medicines, more tests, hearing that mom's blood pressure has been too high, that she fell twice more at night trying to go to the bathroom, that she is losing weight and may need supplements, and that the doctor thinks she needs a psychiatrist consult for her confusion and agitation. Some calls come early in the morning, some of the people calling are barely able to be understood and often have a sense of panic in their voice. Social workers ask more about advanced directives and living wills and finances, while nurses continue to barrage them with every clinical change that occurs. Everyone is trying to help them, and most families know that, but the situation becomes difficult to bear. The level of tension rises, and slowly many family members are dragged into the long-term care zeitgeist where illness is not tolerated, where deterioration needs to be addressed aggressively, where there must be a reason for everything that goes wrong.

Virtually every nurse and social worker with whom I work knows the folly of aggressive care in the frail elderly. It often upsets them to have to be party to the assault. Very often, early in a patient's stay, the staff meets with families and discusses the benefit of palliation. Social workers offer forms that help families move down a path of less aggression.

But families become confused within the contradictory and intense environment that defines long-term care. They are informed about every adverse outcome, every abnormal numerical deviation, every fall and skipped meal. They are often led to believe that they have to choose between aggressive care and death, especially if the specter of hospice is evoked. Often they reach a point of emotional single-mindedness and believe with enough effort mom will not have to die, a belief that is reinforced by family and friends and by the very ethos of American health care delivery. They resist the palliative approach and demand even more aggressive surveillance and treatment. I have seen this occur even among the frailest of my patients, and among those who explicitly stated that they did not want to be kept alive. Sometimes even the most pleasant and intelligent family members become indignant about their loved one's decline, and lose trust in everyone claiming to be trying to help and palliate their mom. And at that juncture, a reluctant staff has to become equally thorough in the patient's care, and the cycle of aggression accentuates to the point of no return.

Nothing makes the system even more dysfunctional than an indignant or frustrated family member. The nurses are frightened to do anything less than everything. Administrators are on edge. And their loved ones who live in the facility become more anxious and thus get more confused; they act out, eat less, and have higher blood pressure. I have seen stable demented people tossed onto the gurney of an ambulance so many times, due not to their own illness but rather to the stress and thorough care that is smothering them. What should be a comfortable haven becomes a hellish plunge into medical excess for the old and demented residents there.

Take the case of Mrs. S. She was quite demented and lived in the nursing home. She was declining by many parameters. She was more confused, losing weight, having elevations of blood pressure, more shortness of breath, and leg swelling. She screamed out often and was resistant to care, including refusing to eat and not allowing aides to wash or dress her. Her daughters were quite aggressive; in the recent past they had brought her to an army of specialists who flooded her with a ton of medicines, all of which she still took. Now, as per family wishes, we ordered x-rays and blood tests frequently. Several times she was shoved into the hospital when she seemed on the verge of death, or when her vital signs destabilized, and there her debility only accentuated and nothing of value was accomplished. A definitive cause of the decline was not ascertained by even the most thorough testing. Nurses checked daily weights, checked vital signs many times a day, and tried to feed her and persuade her to swallow supplements. All of this only seemed to make her worse. The daughters visited constantly. They tried to push her to eat, to walk, to feel better. They were worried about their mom, whom they loved dearly.

Finally, after many meetings and conversations with doctors, nurses, and social workers, they decided to put their mom on hospice. They did not want her in a hospital again or to be artificially fed (something reflected in her living will), and they were told that with her decline, hospice was the only viable option. After much hand-holding and reassurance, the daughters agreed to stop their mom's medicines and to keep her comfortable. No more blood tests, x-rays, weights, or vital signs were taken. Mrs. S. ate only when and what she wanted.

Within weeks Mrs. S. started to improve. She was brighter, happier, and less confused. She ate much better. Her daughters smiled and laughed with her, instead of fussing over her as they had before, and she clearly enjoyed that. Nurses talked to her and laughed with her, rather than putting on blood pressure cuffs and trying to push food down her throat. She enjoyed that too. She became herself again, talking more, becoming more interactive, and not yelling out.

After a few months of steady improvement, and ultimately the decision by hospice to dismiss Mrs. S. due to the fact she no longer was declining, one of the daughters approached me. "Now that mom is better," she asked, "shouldn't we put her back on her medicines? I am afraid her blood pressure may get too high, and her cholesterol too." I just had to chuckle. She did not get it. Few people do. The medicines and treatments and stress were killing her, not her alleged problems. And now they wanted to instigate the whole cascade all over again.

## The Medicare Trap

As I write this chapter I am grappling with a similar situation, but one that is instigated by Medicare itself. Mrs. R., a pleasant woman from an assisted-living facility who had baseline dementia, suffered a severe stroke that left her paralyzed on her left side, unable to talk, and unable to swallow. The hospital doctor persuaded her daughter to surgically place a feeding tube into her gut with the hope that these bags of liquid nutrition would keep her alive long enough to allow her to recover. The daughter acceded to this, not to prolong her life but rather to buy her some time. She was in the hospital for three days, so she was sent to a nursing rehabilitation unit with a "skilled" status, meaning that Medicare would pay most of the bill as long as she remained skilled.

But Mrs. R.'s condition only deteriorated in the rehabilitation facility. She was stricken with bouts of pneumonia from the liquid nutrition rushing up her esophagus and into her lungs, not an uncommon scenario in tube-fed stroke victims. She developed a painful bedsore on her buttocks from a lack of mobility. Her weakness had given no hint of improving. She could not talk or otherwise express herself. As the weeks progressed, and she became further trapped in a body riddled with discomfort, we could all see a deep sense of hopelessness overtake her.

Mrs. R.'s daughter is reasonable, and she agrees that the time has come to withdraw care, but there is a catch.

As long as Mrs. R. receives tube feeds, Medicare will pay her nursing home bill. She is considered "skilled," which is a ticket punch for payment. But if the feeding is stopped, or if Mrs. R. enrolls in hospice, Medicare A will drop Mrs. R., and the $300 daily nursing home bill falls into her daughter's lap. The daughter came to my office in tears. She wants to pull the tube and set up hospice. But she simply cannot afford it. Medicare will only help her if she acts in a way that she knows is contrary to her mother's wishes and contrary to compassionate care. The system has trapped her.

The "skilled" status that was created by Medicare to enable payment for rehabilitation in a nursing home after a significant illness has become itself a trigger for aggressive care in long-term care. It is far less costly for a long-term care facility to send a sick patient to the hospital rather than treat them in the facility, even if the medical system (and Medicare) has to pay much, much more to treat people in the hospital. Very sick residents exhaust too many resources, making them time drains for nurses and aides, demanding levels of care that are often far too expensive both for the facility and for families. Sick demented residents often do not eat, they need IV fluids and medicines, they act out and refuse care, they scream and bite. Often facilities are forced to ask families to hire private aides for very ill residents, or to agree to pay for the IVs and other extra care that Medicare does not cover, something that is not only very expensive but can irritate a family who is already paying a lot. Once patients go to the hospital and have their tickets punched for three nights, then the family pays less, and the facility gets paid significantly more. True, society has to pay a lot more to send such a patient to the hospital, and it is often the wrong thing to do for an older demented patient, but financial reality trumps common sense; it saves everyone money and relieves nursing homes from stress. To watch an old, frail, and demented patient being put on a gurney and dragged kicking and screaming to a hospital, where he will be exposed to illness and excessive intervention, is painful but understandable given the realities of our reimbursement system.

Take the example of pneumonia and dehydration. I have had nursing home patients who develop pneumonia, but are stable. They are not eating well, but can manage with a lot of help. Sometimes they require intravenous medicine and fluids, something that most facilities can provide, and typically they do need extra care. In fact, studies show that nursing home patients with pneumonia treated in their own beds do as well or better than those sent to the hospital.[358] [359] [360] But Medicare does not pay for extra care in the nursing home or assisted-living facility beyond doctor visits. Facilities would need to devote more nursing and aide time to that one patient, taking it away from all the others. It would have to pay to have people manage intravenous lines, often in patients who pull at the lines and cause bleeding and other complications. The medicines and fluids themselves are very expensive for facility and family alike, a cost not covered by Medicare. Rather than suffer all of that, facilities send such patients to the hospital. The benefits for facility and family are immediately apparent. In the hospital Medicare pays for everything. The facility has one fewer sick person to deal with. The family has fewer bills to pay. And if the patient can stay in the hospital three nights and is skilled, suddenly all those expensive medicines and treatments are paid for and the patient returns to the facility with a punched ticket, saving both the facility and the family even more money. Medicare makes everyone is a winner with aggressive care!

## Shoved into the Hospital

Well, there are two losers. One is the tax paying public who now must foot large Medicare bills to pay for unnecessary and costly hospitalizations. The second is the patient himself, since he will now be exposed to the very dangerous hospital. I have seen so many nursing home residents return from hospitals sicker, more confused, more frail and having more aliments (resistant infections, bed sores, increased weakness, hospital-acquired diarrhea, to name a few) than when they left. It is clearly safer for them to stay in the nursing home and be treated there, be treated by people who know them, and be kept away from tests, restraints, medical mistakes, inactivity and bugs that are common in the hospital setting.

We have already discussed how dangerous hospitals can be for elderly patients. The frail elderly who inhabit nursing homes, especially those with dementia, fare even worse. A recent *New England Journal of Medicine* study concluded that transitions of nursing home patients to hospitals are both burdensome "and of limited clinical value." Patients have an increased risk of feeding tube placement, confusion, inadequate attention to their needs, poor communication, and development of large skin ulcers. Citing the financial pressures that push facilities to send their demented residents to hospitals despite the risks, the study concludes: "Transitions among patients with advanced dementia are often avoidable because common complications in such patients can be treated with equal efficacy in the nursing home."[361] Medical errors are also common in the transition between nursing home and hospital, causing even more trauma to the vulnerable patient.[362] [363] As we have shown already, with hospitalization dementia and functional status worsens, infections increase, and overall condition can decline among the elderly.

Of course it would be far cheaper for Medicare to pay facilities to hire more aides and provide basic services than to allow adverse clinical outcomes to occur in the first place, and to pay for treatment in a facility without having to resort to the hospital-derived skilled status. Aides come cheap (sadly, because they are paid so poorly) and they directly prevent many untoward outcomes, such as falls, bed sores, urinary infections, confusion, anxiety, and the list goes on. But given the current economic realities of nursing home medicine, and given the regulatory environment and the prevailing belief that sick people belong in a hospital, such a change in tactics cannot occur without significant reform.

## Lawyers

The other catalyst to aggression that we have already discussed is legal reality. We have all seen commercials on TV with shady lawyers asking if you or a loved one has suffered from nursing home neglect. The very concept that a nursing home can be sued if a resident suffers a bad outcome is something that most of us have witnessed far too often to simply dismiss. Having felt the sting of a bogus lawsuit personally, I am particularly empathetic to facilities that practice defensive medicine. Why should nursing home administrators keep potential liabilities in their facility, where adverse outcomes are very likely, when they can ship them to hospitals and thus deflect the lawyer's spear? It is always legally prudent to be aggressive, to over treat and over test, and to ultimately dump sick people in the hospital.

The financial cost of nursing home lawsuits is substantial. Concludes one study: "Litigation diverts resources from resident care" due to its excessive cost.[364] Long-term care facilities that try to improve their atmosphere to enhance resident quality, such as by providing a more homelike environment for dementia residents, are susceptible to liability,[365] likely because they do not follow standard procedures and are not as aggressive with traditional medical care. But such creative approaches to dementia care also afford patients more freedom. Such patients may wander into rooms and may even fall. Sometimes they will not shower and will not want to get dressed. Their level of comfort and dignity is much improved, by my observations, and they are less likely to be combative, but from a legal standpoint such patients are facility liabilities.

## The Consequences of Thorough

Many of us who work in long-term care innately comprehend the futility of sending our oldest and frailest patients down the road of thorough. We often talk about it with each other, commiserating about our frustration with a system that encourages us to do too much. I have worked with the most wonderful nurses and social workers, who are underpaid and undervalued given all that they know and do. Every nurse and social worker with whom I have been associated has entered his/her field for the most noble of reasons, always with the objective to help patients and families. That they have to confront vulnerable families with hard decisions about life and death, with regulations and requirements, with an absurd financial reality, and with mounds of frustrating paperwork is a problem not of their own making. That they have to call families with every adverse outcome and offer hospitalization and aggressive treatment as an option is not something that most nurses desire. Given that the default setting of every long-term care institution is glued to thorough care, with hospitalization assumed as the best approach for patients who fall too far out of the acceptable norms, we have a hard time nudging patients and families toward a more palliative approach. It requires too much sweat and counterintuitive persuasion and paperwork; it requires families to make too many difficult decisions all at once. It is far easier for everyone just to go with the default.

I conducted an unofficial survey of how many of my long-term care residents were sent to the hospital during the six weeks that it took to write this chapter. Understand that I do everything I can to avoid hospitalization, that I have a financial incentive to keep them out of the hospital and to see them more frequently in their facility when they are ill, that I have nurse practitioners seeing my patients regularly in facilities in an effort to avert hospitalization, and that I am only one doctor and thus have a fairly small long-term care population. Still, during those six weeks, I had over seventy people sent to the hospital. Most were sent for falls, confusion, high blood pressure, abnormal labs, or breathing problems. More than half were admitted to the hospital, but in my estimation only a handful of those really needed in-hospital treatment. Many returned with infections, were functionally and mentally more impaired, and were no better off than they had been before in regard to the problem for which they were sent. Virtually all of them, even those only spending time in the emergency room, had thousands of dollars of testing and treatment that resolved nothing. Even with the most conservative estimates of fees, the overall cost to Medicare for hospital visits for this six-week slice of my small practice was several hundreds of thousands of dollars. And the cost to the patients, to their quality of life and their functional capacity, was immeasurable.

In our county, certain "hot spots" have been identified in which the hospitalization rate is high. These areas are small geographical slices where substantially more people find themselves in the hospital regularly than anywhere else in the county. What unites the hot spots of

Howard County is that each of them has a long-term care facility within its boundaries, which is where the bulk of hospital admissions originate. Ironically, since I am affiliated with many long-term care institutions in the county, I am likely targeted as a doctor who overutilizes the hospital simply by the hot-spot equation. Thus despite the fact that I aggressively keep people out of the hospital with as much power as I possess, that power pales against the forces in long-term care pushing patients in the other direction. Some reformers believe that I can alter that reality, that if facilities are better educated, that if they call us every time something goes wrong, that if we have a nurse practitioner or doctor available to drive over there at a moment's notice, then hospitalizations can be averted. But that myth flies against the reality of regulations, finances, and attitude; doctors and nurses do not want to hospitalize the frail elderly, and many families deep in their hearts do not want to either, but the system pushes aggression on our laps anyway.

Given the reality of patient and family wishes that favor palliation, one wonders why the current trends cannot be reversed. Ninety-six percent of family members report that comfort is their primary goal. But, as one researcher states: "the pattern of transition among nursing home residents with advanced cognitive impairment is often inconsistent with that goal." A fifth of demented nursing home residents are sent to the hospital, and in some states that number is closer to 40 percent. There is no correlation between patient/family wishes and the number of hospital trips.[366] In another study, 25 percent of long-term care residents were hospitalized at least once during a six-month interval, without correlation to patient/family wishes to avoid hospitalization. "[P]hysically frail patients, who may be the least likely to benefit from hospitalizations, are the most likely to be hospitalized," the study concluded.[367] In another study, 40 percent of hospitalization occurred within three months of nursing home admission, and the rate of hospitalization was 566/1000 resident years.[368]

An aggressive mentality sprouts early in a resident's nursing home stay and can fester as time moves forward and signs of illness manifest. When staff and physicians/NPs have time to discuss the futility of thorough care and the natural decline inherent to aging with patients and families, a small dent can be made in the trend. Facilities with more doctors and nurse practitioners available to see residents and families have fewer hospitalizations, although even those numbers are very high.[369] But many patients and families have not pondered these issues before marching into long-term care, and then are stuck by an atmosphere that pushes them in a direction that may not reflect their wishes. Only 75 percent of adults even have advanced directives,[370] and many of those who have completed living wills have done so in a vacuum where they could not envision many of the decisions they now face. In my state, every resident admitted to a long-term care facility must complete a MOLST form, which is essentially a living will, and for many this is the first time they have pondered such weighty questions. Financial realities and state surveys are two other prime reasons that hospitalization occurs with such high frequency.[371] Families are often blindsided by the long-term care onslaught, although many too have some degree of faith in thorough medical care, which allows them to acquiesce to what is transpiring.

## Hospice

Among the elderly, palliative approaches can decrease pain, shortness of breath, and general discomfort while increasing quality of life and both patient and family satisfaction. There is no proven increased mortality in the elderly population who chose to be palliative. But the idea of hospice and palliative care is frightening to many patients and families. They believe that by accepting comfort care they have to abandon hope and accept that death is inevitable. Such a misconception of palliative care is embedded in Medicare's regulations, since Medicare rules stipulate that people have to be end of life and relinquish disease treatment in order to obtain palliative benefits by enrolling in hospice.[372] In other words, Medicare will only pay for palliative care if a patient is on the verge of death.

Thus to most players in long term care—from providers to administrators to families and patients—the only responsible and financially feasible alternative to excessive care that leads so frequently to hospitalization is that of giving up and preparing for death. Recently I was confronted by a facility nurse forcing me to make a bitter decision that has become quite familiar to me. One of my patients, who is very demented and unstable, fell and hit his head. The facility wanted to send him to the hospital, but his daughter did not want that done. She had come to the conclusion that she wanted her dad to be comfortable. So the nurses told me that the daughter had a choice: either send her dad to the hospital, or enroll him in hospice. This black and white option is something that is thrust at doctors and families almost every day. And at its core is an assumption that if families reject the ethos of aggressive care and hospitalization, then their only other choice is to let their loved one die.

Hospice is a Medicare benefit designed to help people at the end of life, typically for those who have cancer and who are actively dying. Hospice patients can obtain more nursing, extra support, pain medicines, medical equipment, and even a brief stay in a hospice in-patient unit when death is imminent and needs are extensive. Typically patients can receive care in the comfort of their homes or long-term care facilities, fully paid for by Medicare. Hospice provides emotional and physical support. Anyone who has been part of hospice, either as a family member or health care provider, agrees that it is the most wonderful experience they could have had during the most difficult time of their lives. In my experience, hospice has been one of the most forward-thinking and compassionate programs that Medicare ever devised, allowing people to die with dignity and without stress, paying for home care and for appropriate treatments without delay or administrative hurdles, and keeping people out of harm's way when they are most vulnerable. I am lucky to work with several excellent hospice agencies that provide superb care.

While hospice, when appropriately used, helps residents in long-term care die in comfort, hospice can also be something employed by facilities and families as the only crutch they have to keep residents away from aggressive care and to have Medicare foot some of the bill. Once families agree to hospice they essentially declare that they want only comfort and are prepared for death. The hospice agency gets paid quite well by Medicare to provide such a benefit, about $4500 per month per enrollee.[373] One *New York Times* report examined the enrollment of patients in hospice and found that many remained in hospice care for prolonged periods of time, sometimes requiring no or minimal services. During those stints hospice was paid $147-$856/day ($4410/month-$25,680/month) depending on the level of care and "regardless of whether a hospice actually provides service."[374] A more recent *Washington Post* exposé made a similar claim, citing that the number of patients discharged alive from hospice increased by 50 percent between 2002–2012, with an increased average length of stay during that period. The article's authors state that a large number of these patients were not hospice appropriate, and were only enrolled because of the financial remuneration.[375] Perhaps many of these patients were not on the verge of death, but they did not want excessive care. With hospice, they could achieve their goals and get some financial help. Without hospice, hospitalization often becomes the only recourse, since home care and appropriate long-term care are not financially feasible otherwise under Medicare. And perhaps too some of these patients actually clinically improved after being enrolled in hospice, living longer because they were removed from the claws of aggressive care, such as Mrs. S who I discussed earlier.

In many long-term care facilities, then, hospice is a way for the facility to get an albatross off its back. If a family does not buy into the mentality of aggressive care that is expected and assumed, then the family is told that it should enroll its loved one in hospice. Once in hospice, then the facility no longer bears the responsibility to prevent and account for someone's decline. Without the label of hospice, patients are assumed to need to be hospitalized and weighed and monitored and tested routinely, blood pressure and sugars are expected to be tightly controlled, and families are expected to be called incessantly and to pay for extra services that Medicare will not cover. With hospice, some of that expectation and financial burden is expunged.

Certainly, that is not the intent of hospice, but for many families and facilities it is the only palliative option Medicare provides. I always say that the landscape between hospice and aggression is called good geriatric care. This is ground rarely trod upon because it is something that Medicare does not support financially, even though hospice agencies would be ideal vehicles to oversee the delivery of such care. Palliative care, as we have discussed, does not assume that patients are on the verge of death. Rather, it correctly reasons that with medical care focused on comfort and dignity that relies less on number chasing and testing, quality improves for patient and family alike. It is the basic soul of good geriatric health care, especially for the old and frail residents of long-term care facilities. It is the type of care that many hospice agencies would like to deliver if only they could be authorized to do so, and likely at a much lower cost.

Hospice is certainly problematic in several ways, most of which stem from Medicare's suffocating rules. Patients can turn on and off hospice at their whims; they can discharge themselves from hospice and rush to the hospital to get aggressive treatment, followed by a "skilled" rehabilitation stay, and then return to hospice subsequently. They can also continue to see specialists and maintain full code status. Therefore, there is no need for hospice patients to truly adhere to a palliative mindset since Medicare will pay either way. Also, because of its function as an instrument in end of life care, hospice relies heavily on pain management, something not necessarily relevant to the needs of many demented elderly. But most problematic about hospice is its narrow focus. Because admission to hospice is becoming more restrictive, many patients who would benefit from a palliative approach do not qualify for hospice services, and they are thus vulnerable to the jungle of long-term care aggression. While the *New York Times* article I cited points to the high cost of hospice, the truth is that if hospice deflects even a handful of hospital admissions, hospice's cost will translate into a substantial monetary savings for Medicare. By stipulating that hospice can only serve end-of-life patients, Medicare is denying palliative treatment to a large numbers of elders who would benefit from such an approach, and as such is inflicting financial harm on itself by opening the door wide to expensive and ineffective aggressive care.

So no, as wonderful as it is for end-of-life care, hospice is not currently a viable answer to our long-term care mess because it is not sufficiently expansive and is becoming even less of a viable option for many elderly as inclusion criteria narrow amid the increased scrutiny being leveled at hospice admission practices. Recently my ACO chided my patients' high hospice enrollment rate, seeing no difference between the Medicare A funds my patients were spending on hospice and on hospitalization. That of course can be easily repaired if Medicare equates hospice not to end-of-life care but rather to palliative care. Under Medicare's current hospice rules is sewn an assumption that is pervasive in all long-term care: that unless a patient undergoes the type of thorough care manifested by number-chasing, tests, treatments, and hospitalization, then the only other option is death. Either we jump on the train of thorough, which is the default of long-term care, or we enroll patients in hospice and accept that death is inevitable. The middle ground, which is the fertile landscape of palliative geriatric care, has been completely bulldozed away.

## Looking Ahead

The future of long-term care is not necessarily any rosier than what we are seeing now, although Medicare is trying to make some changes, as we will explore in the next chapter. At a recent conference of medical directors (AMDA) held in Maryland, I saw a glimpse of what may lie ahead. Talks by academic leaders, CMS officials, and influential medical directors spelled out a frightening scenario. Long-term care regulations not only are here to stay, but they may become more intense, especially in assisted-living facilities. Penalties for doctors and facilities are escalating, and surveys will likely occur with increasing frequency. Privacy laws (HIPAA) are becoming more tightly regulated in long-term care, leading to more possible fines for facilities and doctors alike. And the very ethos of aggressive treatment seemed to have gained a foothold in this group of very wise geriatric doctors, many of whom spoke about the need to tightly control disease among the frail elderly.

At one of the talks, a group of geriatric leaders from major academic institutions outlined a possible nursing home of the future. One of them talked about how nursing homes may soon be able to offer blood transfusions, aggressive treatments, minor surgeries, and even a hospital level of treatment. In other words, they would keep nursing home residents out of the hospital by essentially transforming nursing homes into hospitals.[376] Somehow reformers have convinced themselves that providing aggressive and intensive care to the frail elderly within the nursing home walls is good medicine.

In the end, long-term care seems to mimic a hospital more every day. Unfortunately, its population is the one most hurt by a hospital level of care. Currently the hospital is a common destination for long-term care residents, who are pushed down a road of aggression far more than they should be. If reforms are going to save Medicare and rescue the patients whom Medicare serves, then we must redefine what it means to deliver quality and compassionate geriatric care instead of inventing new ways to be "thorough."

Nursing homes themselves are being pushed into a corner. Most administrators I know and work with, most nurses and aides, most social workers and physicians are trapped in the web of aggression that has been thrust on us by external forces that we can neither mitigate nor control. We are all cognizant of how the current scenario is contrary to geriatric wisdom. But we have little choice but to comply. The ramifications of simply providing good, compassionate care are far too treacherous to enable us to follow that path.

Current reforms by CMS hope to curb hospitalization, seemingly the most obvious and costly ramification of aggressive care. There are some innuendos in Medicare's programs that alternatives to the three-night rule are being considered, although nothing concrete has been proposed to replace it. One informed speaker at the AMDA conference told us that the three-night rule was here to stay, so I am not convinced that its end is near. More saliently, Medicare is pointing its lens at skilled nursing home residents, devising plans that financially reward and punish hospitals and nursing homes that readmit skilled residents to the hospital within thirty days of their hospital discharge. CMS reasons that substantial cost is incurred by such readmissions. But the program is not without its flaws. Because CMS has handed hospitals the power to administer the global funds to cover the first thirty days of a skilled stay, nursing homes are left in the cold. Very likely hospitals will start building their own subacute units so they can better control the post-hospital window, and this will take from nursing homes their most profitable residents. Also, while Medicare's thirty-day readmission moratorium dissuades facilities from hospitalizing a select group of residents for a brief stretch of time, its payment structure continues to encourage admission outside that window. In fact, for hospitals and nursing homes to reap any financial incentives that Medicare will provide them to avert readmissions, there must first be an initial hospital admission to initiate the process, an irony that obfuscates the program's purpose.

Can nursing homes really prevent hospital readmissions in the current environment? How can one group of residents (skilled patients in the thirty-day window) be treated one way, and all other residents (where hospitalization may be beneficial to the nursing home and hospital alike) be treated differently? Can the modus operandi be turned on and off for different groups of patients that quickly? Also, during that thirty-day window, nursing homes will still be subjected to the same regulations and threats of lawsuits that make aggressive care and hospitalization seem necessary, and thus they can be hurt just as much from not hospitalizing a resident as from hospitalizing her.

As long as the current long-term care culture remains intact, meaningful reform will be nothing but window dressing placed upon one of the most salient drains of Medicare's funds. Without malpractice reform, regulatory reform, and profound alterations of Medicare's payment structure, including the elimination of the three-day rule, long-term care facilities have no realistic capacity to move toward a medically sensible and economically sound mode of care. Facilities do want to make that leap, but they are handcuffed. As we conclude the book, we will discuss current reform efforts and explore other ideas that may help save Medicare from its current quagmire.

# 6

# CURING MEDICARE

*Some argue that placing financial barriers to excessive medical
care favors the wealthy since they can pay for such care while the poor
cannot. But that logic is no different than saying that higher cigarette
taxes favor the rich since they can afford to buy cigarettes while the poor
cannot. Excessive care is dangerous, and society need not be forced to pay
for it. If someone seeks to purchase excessive care on his own, let him be
the fool. But if we choose to purchase it for him, then we are the fools.*

Recently doctors placed a stent in one of President George W. Bush's
heart's blood vessels. Apparently during his annual physical his very
thorough primary care doctor ordered an exercise stress test, which
demonstrated an abnormality. President Bush then had a CT angiogram, followed by a cardiac catheterization and stent of the blocked
vessel. The news media glowed at the medical "save" orchestrated by
President Bush's outstanding doctor. One NPR program reveled at our
former President's care, stating that other patients should demand similar thorough treatment.

But, as a well-argued opinion piece in the *Washington Post* demonstrated, President Bush's stress test was likely unnecessary and was potentially harmful. Stated the physician authors: "If Mr. Bush had visited
a general internist practicing sound, evidence-based care, he would
not have had cardiac testing." At age sixty-seven, our former President

jogged regularly and bicycled long distances all without symptoms or limitations. No study has demonstrated the efficacy of screening stress tests in such a patient, nor has any study shown that stenting the type of occluded artery found during the testing improves either lifespan or life quality. In fact, now President Bush will be at higher risk for having to take two blood thinners to prevent the stent from collapsing and blocking the vessel entirely.[377] Most significantly, President Bush now carries a diagnosis of coronary artery disease (CAD), a label that will define him for the rest of his life; lead to more tests, procedures, medicines, and specialist visits down the road; and may even impact him psychologically. Worse still, while it is unclear whether Medicare would pay for the initial stress test given to President Bush and patients like him, it certainly would pay for all subsequent testing and the placement of the stent, and it would continue to pay for all cardiac testing, specialist visits, and further stenting for as long as our President , or any other Medicare recipient, lives. One test ordered in the name of thorough instigated a cascade of further testing and treatments, all without proven benefit, all with potential harm, and yet Medicare paid without blinking an eye, and the news media praised the wonderful medical care.

President Bush is only sixty-seven. Many of my patients who are much older certainly have blocked arteries. If we look hard enough we will find them, and we can send them too on a similar expensive and precarious course that is financed by Medicare and cheered by society and the lay press. But we also have evidence that such aggressive treatment is not medically beneficial to our oldest patients, and may actually be deleterious. Even as our society scoffs at the high cost of Medicare, it ignores the simple fact that Medicare is enabling and even encouraging our costly trek through a wilderness of inappropriate medical care for the frail elderly. In fact, much of society considers such care both necessary and thorough.

An excellent illustration of this relates to skin cancer. We are always being told to inspect our skin and to look out for cancers. Some cancers are deadly (melanoma especially), others are less likely to kill or maim. In my older patients the nonlethal skin cancers (squamous cell and basal cell carcinomas) are fairly ubiquitous, sometimes littering their bodies. Years of sun exposure takes its toll. I always inspect my patient's skin but I am rarely alarmed, even if I suspect a cancer, unless the lesion is growing, causing discomfort, or demonstrates worrisome features. But when my patients decide to visit dermatologists, those bumps suddenly take on an urgency and must be excised immediately, sometimes requiring surgical eradication. A recent study estimates that 2.2 million Americans are diagnosed with nonmelanoma skin cancers annually, mostly older people in the Medicare age group. These cancers are typically slow growing and do not impact survival or quality of life. Still, most had the lesions removed, and 20 percent of the older patients reported a significant complication of the procedure, including poor wound healing, numbness, and pain. Still, despite the potential harm and the lack of demonstrable efficacy, it is recommended that all such lesions be removed.[378] Dermatologists are well paid for their thorough "life-saving" procedures; Medicare pays the bill, and the lay press touts how important it is to get regular skin checks and cure those skin cancers. But are our patients better off to have been exposed to a surgical procedure with no demonstrable impact on mortality or quality of life, even though most think and are told that their lives were saved and their federally financed insurance will blindly pay?

A recent *New York Times* article from January 2014 explored the explosion of dermatology procedures in this country for often nonlethal lesions. The article cites the lucrative nature of skin biopsies for the doctors performing them, and the atmosphere of fear that has been inculcated into our thinking making us all believe that biopsies and radical skin cancer eradication are essential and lifesaving.[379] The truth of such claims is questionable, skin cancer treatment is likely being overutilized, patients are harmed, and Medicare funds are being needlessly squandered. But nothing is being done to stop the process, and in fact more doctors and patients are buying into this aggressive model of care.

When we examine why Medicare is going broke we do not have to look much beyond the skin. The perception that we should be looking for and eradicating every disease process in our older patients is the very root of Medicare's demise. It is a myth that is inscribed into the very soul of Medicare itself, as Medicare is focused on finding and fixing diagnoses and numbers rather than helping people to age well and feel better. Many Americans understand that Medicare is wasteful, but few are willing to acknowledge from where such waste emanates. Any restriction of unnecessary care is labeled as rationing, and that word has doomed all past attempts at health care reform.

In this country many reform efforts are hampered by what I call the Katrina effect. In Louisiana, the governor and many of the politicians have always touted a "get the government off our backs" philosophy that is endemic in many areas of our country. Yet when Hurricane Katrina massacred its shores, suddenly the governor and other Gulf State politicians demanded immediate and expansive federal aid, criticizing the federal response as being inadequate. Years later, when just as devastating a storm struck New Jersey, those same politicians voted against aid to the state, claiming that the federal government simply could not afford it. That is the Katrina effect. We are all against the government's out-of-control spending, but if we need the funds, we want it immediately and without limitations. The effect has a profound impact on Medicare reform efforts and is the primary reason that rationing is such a bedeviled word. While we all want to curb Medicare spending, we want to personally be able to utilize as many Medicare resources that we think we or our family members need, despite the cost or proven efficacy.

And yet, we all know that Medicare reform must occur. Currently, as we have said, much of Medicare's dollars flow to the sickest and oldest of our patients without any proof that such money improves quality or length of life. Much of that is spent for end-of-life care, where huge expenditures are squandered in situations with tragic outcomes. Why is not the bulk of our reform effort aimed at reducing that number? Is it because so many people and organizations—doctors, hospitals, medical supply companies, pharmaceuticals—financially prosper from our current aggressive health care landscape that spends money without regard to meaningful outcomes? Is it because American society and its politicians truly believe that all people, regardless of their prospects for survival, deserve the full gamut of aggressive medical care before they are allowed to die? Or is it because, by eschewing alternatives to such care such as palliative and home-based services, Medicare has left us no other options?

Certainly the Katrina effect is at play; we may theoretically believe that it is wasteful for the system to spend a quarter of its budget on ineffective care, while we still want mom to be given everything modern health care can throw at her at the end of her life, primarily because we never are willing to admit it is the end; our faith in the American medical system tell us that with enough effort we can achieve the impossible. Also, many Americans believe that since they have put money into Medicare during their working lives, they deserve all the medical care they desire; after all, they paid for that care. Unfortunately, since the average American spends $387,000 of Medicare money during his/her lifetime, and has only contributed $88,000 to Medicare,[380] society is paying for the vast majority of the excessive and wasteful care that Medicare is both allowing and encouraging.

## Models of Change

Interestingly, in our own country, we do have a government-financed health care system that does put limitations on care and yet produces excellent health outcomes and high patient satisfaction for some of the sickest patients in the system. This is our Department of Veterans Affairs (VA), where patients have limited specialty access, ample primary care, a strict drug formulary, and services geared to help the specific patient population being served.[381] The VA is certainly not free of its own difficulties, not the least of which are a growing reliance on clinical performace measures and a shortage of primary care doctors at times (leading to longer wait times, and endemic of the primary care shortage that grips our entire nation), but it achieves quality care for patients at a low cost. Also, the VA is always innovating. With expansive home care services, specialty consultations that do not require a visit, and the ability of doctors to "visit" patients at their homes through telephone and computer technology, the VA is able to achieve its goals without having to resort to as much specialization and hospitalization. Medicare, with its strict rules about paying doctors only for face-to-face visits and procedures, will not permit this efficient and effective model of care.

Another current innovative strategy that has been enacted in this country for several decades relies on capitated health care plans called health maintenance organizations (HMOs). Medicare HMOs are insurance companies of varying sizes that are paid a specified global fee by Medicare per patient (capitation) and are expected to take full care of that patient—including all hospitalizations, doctor visits, and procedures—for that amount of money. If the companies can treat their cohort of patients for less money than Medicare pays them, they win financially. If not, they lose. Therefore, HMOs work hard to provide sensible, efficient care.

Unfortunately, despite their promise of providing efficient and cost-effective health care through the free market, HMOs have not made a significant dent in our Medicare crisis. During their history HMOs have proven to be unpopular among many patients because they are perceived to restrict patient choice,[382] thus insinuating that they ration care. Therefore, they have tended to attract the healthiest patients who spend the least amount of health care dollars. Also, studies have demonstrated that HMOs do not curtail doctor visits, or even reduce the cost of end-of-life care.[383][384] Probably the most significant limitation of managed care is that it has never had enough traction to really make an impact. Now more Medicare HMOs are emerging, but under the ACA the current 14 percent subsidy that Medicare pays to HMO venders will be eliminated (see note 7), leaving Medicare HMOs with an uncertain future.

While working at a retirement community I had the opportunity to be part of an HMO that was constructed and piloted by the lead physicians of the community. It was never a large endeavor, and I was not privy to whether it achieved real financial success even with Medicare's 14 percent subsidy, but from my perspective it did work. We eliminated the three-day rule, allowing us to treat patients in our nursing home and in their homes without resorting to hospitalization. Nurses followed patients at home, and primary care doctors made most crucial decisions. Patients still had unfettered access to specialists, tests were not restricted, and clinical practice guidelines retained too much importance, but compared to standard Medicare, the HMO did allow us to take care of our patients in a more humane, sensible fashion. Any model for health care reform should reflect what we have learned from HMOs.

Currently many reformers absorb the lesson of HMOs and reach what I believe to be an erroneous conclusion. They assume that if physicians are paid for their performance rather than for each visit and procedure, then physicians will be incented to provide more efficient, low-cost care and keep elderly patients out of the hospital. This approach is rife with problems. First, it assumes that physicians can influence the specific care that their patients pursue, even if patients are intent on leaping onto the thorough train and are often pushed in that direction. Specialization, the threat of lawsuits, long-term care regulations, and a belief among Americans that more care is better care all will not simply disappear under a pay for performance approach. Thus, primary care doctors cannot impact the aggressive medical environment in which we all live, and cannot alter the course their patients pursue. Second, if primary care doctors are paid to provide less care, then they will certainly be vulnerable to the accusation that they are curtailing care to earn more money, which is a serious conflict of interest. Any good lawyer could use that against a doctor in a liability case, and the jury would eat it up.

In addition, it is very unclear how performance will be defined under a pay for performance model. Clearly performance cannot be equated with how infrequently our patients are hospitalized and tested, since those events occur independently of our own efforts as long as patients retain the ability to control their own health care provision. Thus plans such as Medicare have adapted another more specious approach. Under such proposed systems, physician performance is typically defined by clinical performance measures, which as we have discussed do not reflect true quality geriatric care. If we aggressively treat diabetes, control blood pressure, treat heart disease patients with statins, order bone density tests, and allow open access to specialty care, then our performance is deemed to be of high quality. Thus, those of us who practice good geriatric care are going to be labeled as poor performers under any system using clinical guidelines.

Reformers also are employing a strategy, used by some local hospitals and insurance systems today, that focuses on education to curtail hospitalization. For those patients hospitalized frequently or who spend large amounts of money for their care, care coordinators will help them navigate the medical landscape. Social workers and nurses will guide such patients through the health care delivery system, assisting them with doctor appointments, self-care, and education. Some small studies have shown a cost savings from such a model as well as a reduction in hospital readmission in the first thirty days after discharge.[385] However, such programs are in their infancy and their true utility is yet to be seen.

Another idea being tossed around is to push the Medicare eligibility age up to 67. The thought is that by eliminating a few years of Medicare enrollees from the insurance market, Medicare can instantly save money. But such a concept ignores what we know both about the demographics of aging and the projected spending pattern of Medicare recipients. Most of Medicare's money is spent on our oldest citizens, a group of people whose numbers are expanding rapidly. In fact, the cost savings by denying younger Medicare patients access to insurance would barely dent our pending Medicare crisis. The goal of all reform must focus on the oldest patients, not the youngest, especially those most frail and at the end of their lives.

## Novel Forms of Medicare Reform

Currently multiple reform efforts are being proposed and instituted to help save Medicare from its accelerating state of financial peril. Many are emanating from the government through Medicare's "innovation center"[386] and the Affordable Care Act (ACA).[387] As a practicing physician I have been bombarded by a host of new rules and regulations. Some are so poorly explained to me that I am forced to pay consultants to walk me through the process. Some are so poorly executed that they simply are not possible to carry out. I have been to conferences, read articles, and have talked to CMS experts in an effort to stay one step ahead, often to no avail.

On a very basic level, new ACA and Medicare regulations seem to be targeting home health and home medical equipment, both of which help keep my patients out of the hospital and away from aggressive care. Medicare currently pays only for very limited services at home for brief durations, and the home health nurses with whom I work talk about copious new restrictions that limit the scope of what they can do for my older patients. For me, I now have tremendous paper work requirements to initiate and retain home health services, and to order home medical equipment, especially more expensive items such as electric wheelchairs (which still cost Medicare less than a day in the hospital) and even manual wheelchairs and hospital beds. I now spend over an hour a day filling out the pile of forms that are tossed on my desk primarily related to home health and medical equipment. While the burdens of paperwork have accentuated for home care, I have encountered no such barriers to sending patients to hospitals or specialists and ordering expensive tests. Those remain easy to execute under the ACA and Medicare!

The financial burden to our practice from government initiated regulations and reforms like the new home health rules has been substantial. But other measures are even more costly. For instance, to comply with the electronic medical record requirement we have had to pay for increasingly costly software, pay an IT expert to provide ongoing services, and set up expensive security measures, as well as buying computers and hardware with regularity. Also, given that there is feasible speculation in the medical community that some of the ACA will be financed by auditing doctor offices and fining those whose billing and charting practices do not comply with Medicare standards,[388] [389] I have taken out both coding and HIPAA insurance plans, both of which are costly. Although I believe that I am coding correctly and do not commit HIPAA violations, I can easily envision an auditor finding a few subjective problems that could cost our practice tens of thousands of dollars in fines, if not more.

Recently my HIPAA and Coding insurer dropped me, citing the fact that auditors (who are paid a certain percentage of the fines they levy at doctors, giving them great incentive to escalate the fines) are now targeting geriatric doctors who care for patients in long-term care facilities or who make home visits. I immediately wrote to my congressman and senators. I expressed my outrage at the ACA, a bill I supported, but which now seemed to be strangling primary care. I cited the cost and fear of audits, the cost of electronic records, the increasing regulatory burdens of HIPAA and of required adherence to copious clinical guidelines that are often irrelevant to our patients, the increasing paper work and the inability to provide patients with home health care and with simple medical equipment, the introduction of new billing codes (ICD-10) that are burdensome and time-consuming, and the incessant threat of arbitrary reimbursement cuts coupled with a demand for more accountability. My congressman's staffer did call me back, and we spoke for twenty minutes; she seemed sympathetic but did not seem optimistic that there would be change. My two senators simply did not respond. All three supported the ACA, and all three pay lip service to the need for more primary care in this country. But at present, those two goals are contradictory.

Several weeks later our practice was audited. We were asked to provide forty charts to a CMS contractor. Our sin: that we billed too many codes for seeing people in assisted-living facilities, where many of our patients reside. I spoke to people in CMS, to consultants, to insurance brokers. We read through the forty charts to assess if we had documented everything correctly. We knew that even one missing line from the CMS template would be considered fraud. Although most of the notes seemed extensively documented, none were perfect, and anything less than perfect is potentially considered overpayment. The process was frightening and time-consuming. In the end we came through with flying colors, but we also know that more audits lay ahead. With all the extraneous work Medicare's reforms have tossed on our laps, all the extra cost it has inflicted upon us, it seems that Medicare has decided that it is easier to assault small geriatric primary care practices than to have the resolve to fix a broken system. I wrote again to my senators. And yet again, they did not respond.

We in primary care have received a 10 percent bonus to our Medicare revenue, and we can receive additional bonuses if we comply with electronic medical record standards and participate in our ACO (which we will discuss). But we have had to pay so much more than that to adhere to the accentuating regulations and punitive audits being carried out in the name of innovative reform. My front staff also has to spend large amounts of time contending with the increased paperwork and other requirements stemming directly from reform, something else that adds more cost to our overhead and takes away the time they have to help our patients. We have to hire consultants and other aides to assist us through the complicated web of reforms and changes being thrust at us but which none of us can fully comprehend and no one from Medicare can fully explain. None of this is helping to make primary care a more palatable field, and from what I can see none of it will make any dent in Medicare's pending financial collapse or in our ability to care for elderly patients.

The *New York Times* article cited above with regard to skin cancer reiterates what so many other people have been stating, and what I explored in this book. The dearth of primary care, and the explosion of specialization in our medical society, has led to a procedure oriented culture that is sucking Medicare's funds away without providing any proven medical benefits, something even more apparent for the oldest of our patients. The income of procedure oriented specialists has increased dramatically over the past decade, while primary care income has trickled up modestly, something typically erased by the increased regulatory burdens to which we are forced to adhere. Dermatologists, who perform the biopsies we discussed above, previously earned an income similar to primary care doctors, but now are the fourth-highest paid specialty and have one of the lightest workloads according to the *Times* article. In my opinion, primary care has the opposite profile: the lowest paid, and one of the highest workloads. Despite the talk of government reform and the promises of the ACA, aggressive, specialized medicine will continue to dominate the medical landscape as long as it is well compensated and is not discouraged. Ironically, although the news media often run stories such as the one about dermatology that expose major problems in our current health care delivery system, they also run articles and stories that nudge patients into an aggressive mindset, not the least of which is that patients need annual skin checks and frequent skin biopsies or else they will die of skin cancer, something portrayed as an epidemic in our society. So even while the media blast dermatologists and Medicare for their procedure oriented focus, they implore people to be wary of cancer and to be sure to get those very procedures. Reform cannot work as long as we live in a society that thrives on excess.

I will discuss a few of the government-sponsored reforms that have arrived or are on the way. I will say that I know many people, doctors and others, who work in CMS trying to make Medicare sensible and financially solvent. Their ideas are often quite bold, and they do comprehend many of the issues that thwart Medicare's ability to carry out its primary mission in helping the elderly. But politics, bureaucracy, and vested interests hamper even the most idealistic reformer from applying pragmatic repairs to what we all know to be a broken system. Like me, those I know in CMS believe in Medicare and know that it can be better. Within the tight boundaries of their roles in CMS, they have started to script some fixes, some of which have not been successful in the eyes of a primary care doctor like me, and others that perhaps do hold some potential.

**Electronic Medical Records:** I have worked with Electronic Medical Records (EMRs) for well over a decade, and began my new practice with computers, laptops, and medical software. Without a doubt, the EMR caused me more stress and consternation during my first year in solo practice than anything else. After spending weeks setting up the system, it continuously crashed, always at the least opportune times. I used to stay up past midnight completing my notes and fighting a system that refused to cooperate. After a great waste of dollars and time, and after consulting various experts who often only made matters worse, we stabilized our medical record system, although we still have serious problems on a regular basis. So much can go wrong that likely it will; but after so many years of regular crashes and Internet failures we have finally accommodated to it. It is still where most of us squander the bulk of our time; we are typically in front of the computer more than we are in front of our patients, and even when we are with patients we are focused on typing our scripted notes in exactly the format Medicare demands of us, something that clearly distracts from the doctor-patient encounter.

Medicare does pay for us to certify our medical records, but the stipend, while substantial (approximately $20,000 for initial certification, more incrementally later) costs us a great deal of time, money, and frustration. I spent approximately 40 hours fulfilling the many checklists that CMS mandates to prove my compliance with its EMR requirement, and that is for only part one of the process. And the Medicare stipend does not come close to paying all of the expenses that go into initiating and maintaining an EMR. Technology is our biggest overhead cost, other than salaries.

Medicare and the ACA both tout EMRs as being crucial to health care reform. Perhaps in the future EMRs will help us all be connected: doctor to doctor, doctor to hospital, patient to doctor, lab to doctor and patient. Very little of that is occurring now, and with HIPAA hovering over all of us like a voracious vulture, I cannot imagine connectivity being a very substantial force in the near future. So at this point, EMRs allow us to write notes, send prescriptions, and print/fax orders, that is all. By 2015 all participating Medicare physicians will be required to have an EMR.

How successful are EMRs? They have saved the VA system money. But in the world of private practice, no such financial remuneration has been seen. A 2005 RAND study predicted that EMRs may save the system $81 billion annually. By 2013, however, no health care savings have yet occurred. In fact, some suggest that EMRs actually increase test ordering and thus cost.[390][391] They also allow doctors to increase the billing for their services and possibly charge more for visits. And of course, they divert physician time and resources away from patient care and toward note-taking and computer tinkering. Likely the EMRs will be an important component of modern medicine, but at this juncture they are neither helping the quality of geriatric care nor are they saving the system any money. In fact, they are really just very sophisticated headaches!

**Physician Quality Reporting System (PQRS):** An important mission of CMS is to assure that Medicare doctors practice quality geriatric care, as we discussed extensively in chapter 1. I am speculating that in the future a large chunk of our pay will be determined by our compliance with quality indicators, and some of that is already starting through PQRS. PQRS is simply a means of persuading Medicare physicians to adhere to a specified set of clinical guidelines. When CMS built its PQRS system, it offered a small incentive to those who complied. Now, physicians will suffer reimbursement cuts if they do not comply. Quality is measured by many parameters, and physicians can dig deep into websites and thick books to find specific clinical practice guidelines that can be followed and documented electronically to satisfy Medicare's PQRS requirement. Or physicians can hire and pay a company to provide templates for certain grouped quality measures, survey a small number of patients using the template, and submit the templates electronically to the company, which will forward them to CMS. I chose the latter method and have picked preventive care as my theme. I ask my chosen patients about smoking and drinking, their weight, immunization, mammograms and bone density screening, and colonoscopies. I document this in the chart. Then I fill out papers and submit them. It is time-consuming and costly, but it allows me to demonstrate that I have provided "quality" medical care as defined by clinical performance measures. While I laud CMS for trying to enhance quality, I am not quite sure how this particular reform measure will help improve real geriatric quality, especially given the parameters on which we are being judged. In fact, many of us in primary care cite Medicare's quality indicator requirements as one of the most wasteful and time-consuming endeavors in which we are being forced to participate.

**Accountable Care Organizations (ACOs):** Perhaps the most promising, if perplexing, concept created by the ACA are ACOs, voluntary HMO-like entities that doctors and/or institutions join in an effort to cut cost and improve quality. The basic premise of ACOs is to encourage doctors/hospitals to combine forces and utilize care coordination, clinical practice guidelines, and enhanced communication to decrease the wasteful consumption of care. The ACO will then work as a large unit and its success will be judged by CMS against prevailing standards. States a *Forbes* summary: "The providers in an ACO are responsible for management and care of the health plan enrollees and are financially rewarded if the enrollees or patients stay out of the more expensive hospital."[392]

At least, that is the theory.

I belong to an ACO called Northern Maryland Collaborative Care. One day earlier this year I received a letter and email asking me to join and describing the general philosophy of Accountable Care Organizations, something I had read about at length but did not fully understand. Essentially I would be working with a large group of unnamed doctors and hospitals in my region in an unspecified manner to somehow reduce cost. By joining, I would not relinquish any component of my current relationship with Medicare; my payments would not change for seeing patients, the rules would not change, and the entire care structure would remain intact. According to the provider handbook, ACOs could be composed of professionals in a group practice, networks of individual practices, hospital-professional partnerships, or hospitals that employ professionals, as long as the named group cares for at least 5000 Medicare enrollees and follows a basic organizational structure that the handbook elucidates. In addition, the handbook states that if any of my patients sign up, they too would not lose any of their current benefits or be subject to any new restrictions. States the handbook: "Simply put, there is no change to Medicare benefits whether a patient uses a physician participating in the ACO or not." Patients would be contacted by care coordinators if they did join, both to conduct an initial health assessment and to identify high-risk patients who may need additional services, especially after being in the hospital. The primary goal is to avert future hospitalizations.[393] Not sure what my role in this ill-defined group may be, but assured that I would not be penalized for joining, I signed up.

Since I joined, three things have happened. First, a representative of the ACO came to my office and spent a day collecting the names and other information of all of my Medicare patients. The representative has returned a few other times, and as nice as she is, she has not fully elucidated what my role would be in the ACO process or even who else had joined the ACO. I have also communicated with and met with the ACO executive director to help clarify what is expected of me, including writing annual wellness notes, providing data to the ACO, and adhering to specified clinical guidelines that mimic and expand upon what PQRS is requiring of me. I certainly have not seen any evidence of increased communication among members, or any hint of care coordination, although these elements may come later. I was chided for having too many of my patients on hospice, something I thought was a Medicare benefit that the patients themselves had chosen, and something that has kept many of my most frail patients out of the far more expensive hospital. Second, the ACO representative gave me a check for somehow already having saved money. Again, I am not sure why, although I did take the check and have received a few others since. Third, all of my patients received letters asking them whether they wanted to join the ACO. They received a subsequent letter asking them to rate our practice and me as a doctor. I have spent the last few months trying to explain to my patients—both in the context of talks and patient visits—what joining may entail, essentially telling them that they had very little risk if they joined. Still, many of them are very wary of signing up, especially after they received the survey letter.

Recently I have read and heard more about ACOs, and am not sanguine that I am part of an organization that really will impact the health care crisis, as much as I hope I am wrong. At the AMDA conference in March several talks about ACOs only further confused me, although I did learn that they would become required for all doctors in several years.[394] A *Washington Post* article in July confirmed another fact, which is that as the program is being phased in, doctors will start to be penalized for poor "quality" performance. A doctor's quality grade will be based on his adherence to the very clinical guidelines we have already discussed, and by how much each ACO's average patient costs the system.[395]

Being judged on quality measures that are not patient specific and that often verge from true quality geriatric care drives a dagger of consternation through my gut. According to the handbook in my ACO, quality measures include surveys in which patients not only rate us but are also asked if they retain good access to specialists, essentially assuring that the concept of specialization is encouraged by the ACO. We will also be judged by preventive screening, such as making sure our patients get mammograms; the use of certain medicines in specific cardiac conditions, such as using the heart drugs in patients with CHF that are considered standard of care, and Warfarin in elderly patients with A-fib, despite how those drugs may negatively impact our frail patients; and our ability to control cholesterol, diabetes, and blood pressure by specified parameters and regardless of any other confounding medical issues that may render such control dangerous or ill-advised.[396] In other words, our success will be ascertained by definitions of quality that I have spent this entire book debunking. According to a *JAMA* study, the thirty-three quality measures being employed by ACOs do not have a clear correlation to a population's health. In fact, the study concludes that the overall ACO structure lacks the incentives and structure to really improve a population's overall health as it does not focus on long-term determinants of outcome for the elderly.[397]

For me in particular, another ironic twist is built into the ACO grading system. Since we are judged by how often our patients are hospitalized, and since so many of my patients are in assisted-living facilities, which in our county are hot spots of hospitalization, I may emerge as one of the most egregious hospitalizers in the entire ACO. By not altering the rules of long-term care, and by not making assisted-living facilities partners in the ACO process, health care reformers have provided absolutely no incentive for those facilities to avert hospitalization, something that the current Medicare and regulatory system both encourages and finances. Also, there is nothing built into the ACO model that incentivizes patients and families to stay out of the hospital. In fact, since the ACO concept has not dismantled the three-day rule, has not enabled Medicare financed home based services, and has retainined the extant Medicare reimbursement system that rewards specialization and hospitalization, just the opposite is true. Thus, my patient population will likely continue to flock to the hospital, something that is completely out of my control but is now something for which I will be held accountable. I suppose that is why this is considered accountable care!

And that is an egregious flaw of the entire ACO concept. The ACO contends that tossing a few dollars at doctors and hospitals will entice us to spend less of the Medicare budget on expensive care. But we are not the ones who drive the aggressive model of medical care that is endemic to this country. All they have done is to drop more regulations and penalties into the laps of overburdened primary care doctors. By not addressing the financial realities that drive patients into a hospital instead of being cared for at home, by not assessing true measures of quality, ACOs ask us to do less while not altering the landscape that pushes everyone to do more.

In addition, by not changing the infrastructure of health care delivery and by not altering how doctors are paid, ACOs are trying to accomplish what HMOs could not without having any power to alter the behavior of those who benefit from a more specialized and aggressive health care model. As one observer concludes, the current model "works against the very design of the program. The inequities of the fee-for-service system, which rewards procedural-ists and specialists at the expense of cognitive specialties and pri-mary care, remain embedded in the payment system."[398] In the old HMO model, especially the one I so revered at the retirement com-munity where I worked, primary care doctors ran the show, absurd concepts like the three-day rule were eliminated, home health was better financed and made more creative, and patients had some skin in the game since they received more services if the Medicare Advantage plan saved money. None of this is true in ACOs. States one study done at the inception of the ACO model, "Primary care physicians have little direct leverage over other providers in the care continuum, and under the largely fee-for-service payment system it is unlikely other providers will respond to reductions in the number of referrals or admissions by allowing their incomes to fall." Also, the success of ACOs is limited by the concern that "hospitals and specialists would garner a disproportionate share of any savings."[399]

Although the ACO model relies on care coordination by nurses and social workers to nudge patients down a more sensible clinical path away from the hospital, that idea has proven to be more expensive and complicated than anticipated, especially given the lack of primary care doctors who have time to help facilitate the process.[400] While care coordination is a worthy and potentially beneficial goal, it cannot by itself dam the flow of aggression that dominates our health care delivery system. To advise patients to stay out of the hospital, but then have nothing else to offer them in the way of home and palliative care, deprives care coordinators from truly making a dent in Medicare's flawed payment model. ACOs represent a noble and thoughtful idea, but one without any teeth in the landscape of geriatric health care delivery.

**Bundled Payment System:** Another potentially promising innovation is that of bundled payments, a concept driven by hospitals that is designed to reduce the cost of post-hospital care and curtail the high rate of hospital readmissions from long-term care facilities. It is due to be fully enacted in 2019. Bundled payment systems are a rendition of Diagnostic Related Groups (DRGs) that Medicare codified in 1982 and that have shaped hospital spending ever since. Under DRGs hospitals are paid a certain bundled fee for each diagnosis with which a patient presents, despite how long a patient stays in the hospital for that diagnosis. Medicare has devised 467 diagnostic groups for which it will always pay a set fee.[401] Bundled payments take this concept a step further. Now hospitals will be paid a set fee for both the acute hospital stay AND all services that are required thirty days after the hospital stay, including rehabilitation stints, home health, and even rehospitalization. The goal of bundling patients is to encourage hospitals to identify patients who are at high risk of being readmitted to the hospital and to manage them better to avoid readmissions. Currently it is believed that up to 20 percent of patients are readmitted to the hospital within thirty days of discharge, a high cost to the system. Bundling will incentivize hospitals to cut down this number.[402] I will note that in my patient population, readmissions constitute a very small percentage of overall admissions, and certainly are nowhere near the 20 percent that is cited. Of the large number of hospital admissions that occurred in my long-term patients during the six-week period I was tracking those numbers (see chapter 5), only one or two were readmissions. Thus in my world, bundled payment would impact a very tiny proportion of total hospitalizations.

In fact, in a perverse way, bundled payments may *encourage* hospitalization. Without hospitalizing patients in the first place, hospitals and their contracted agents (physicians, home health services, nursing homes, etc.) will never see the profits that bundled care promises. And after their thirty-day post-hospital stint, it certainly makes financial sense to hospitalize patients again to initiate another bundle. As one study stated, "in an effort to maintain income levels that are necessary to cover fixed costs, providers may change their behaviors to increase the volume of episodes." "Episodes," here, refers to hospitalizations.[403] Bundling payments could also be medically deleterious to patients by denying them certain facets of care (in an effort to cut cost) in the post-hospital period. In fact, the real incentive is not to help the patient have better long-term outcomes, but rather to do well enough in the thirty-day post-hospital period so that they stay out of the hospital for that brief stretch of time. One study states that bundling "in some instances could produce unintended consequences that would contribute to avoidable poor outcomes" among the vulnerable elders,[404] especially when it comes to their long-term outcomes.

At the AMDA conference I attended in March, many of the talks highlighted how bundling will impact the long-term care setting. Currently the program is very limited in scope, but it will expand over the years to include many more diagnoses. In one of the talks, the hospital-affiliated lecturer stated that hospitals could profit from bundled care,[405] and in fact doctors and hospitals are flocking to partake in bundled payments because they are so potentially profitable.[406] It is fairly easy to keep people out of the hospital for thirty days by implementing more aggressive post-hospital services and care coordination. ACE (Acute Care for the Elders) units in hospitals are already accomplishing that goal without the allure of bundling.[407] After thirty days, of course, then it is business as usual; hospitalization is again encouraged, since Medicare no longer pays for the services needed to keep people out of the hospital, and both patients and institutions financially benefit from another hospital stay.

Bundling does not erase many of the ingredients that trigger hospitalization in the first place. The three-day rule will still exist, meaning that facilities and patients both will profit if a patient stays in the hospital for three nights. Also, the current liability and regulatory environment will not be repaired, both of which encourage hospitalization and aggressive care. Virtually every factor we discussed that drives the excessive use of hospitalization among the frail elderly will be left intact outside of the thirty-day window; as with ACOs, bundling payments does not alter the basic skeleton of our health care delivery system that pushes patients to embrace specialization and hospitalization. I am also skeptical of any reform effort that is controlled by the hospital itself. That seems to be a very backward method of reducing hospitalization!

**The Independent Payment Advisory Board (IPAB):** One stipulation of the ACA is the initiation of a payment advisory board that will help guide Medicare policy and recommend pay scales for physicians. The IPAB, which is very controversial among politicians, is a fifteen-member independent panel appointed by the president and confirmed by the Senate. The members are supposed to be nationally recognized experts in health finance, payment, economics, and actuarial science. There is no stipulation that any doctors sit on the board, and certainly no expectation that practicing doctors like me would even be invited. The Board would be able to instigate changes in Medicare with limited congressional input.[408]

A war of words has been bouncing on the Internet regarding the potential impact of the IPAB. Howard Dean, a physician, former governor, and chairman of the DNC, states that similar rate-setting programs have a forty-year track record of failure. Such a Board will not cut costs, he contends. He also points to a perceived flaw of the Board: that a top-down approach to health care reform will not be well accepted: "patients and physicians get aggravated because bureaucrats…are making medical decisions without knowing the patient."[409] Peter Orszag, who helped to create the IPAB, counters that the Board is necessary to guide Medicare into a new era. The Board, he states, will be "tweaking our evolving payment system in response to incoming data and experience…"[410]

From all we know about Medicare reform and what needs to be accomplished, it is hard to imagine that a group of politically appointed "experts" who have no firsthand experience with the practice of medicine will be able to transcend their parochial perceptions and create a sensible health care delivery system for seniors. Unless practicing primary care physicians are involved in crafting reform, the result is likely to be a complicated, formulaic strategy that misses the point. As I have suggested throughout this book, we in primary care know what is wrong with Medicare and how to save it. We understand why current policy will not be effective, for many of the reasons I have elucidated. And we know what barriers stand in the way. The only problem we have is that no one ever asks us.

**The Medicare Innovation Center (CMMI):** With a staff of nearly three-hundred employees, and a budget of ten billion dollars over ten years, the CMMI is a part of the ACA designed to finance projects initiated in the medical community that will improve quality care and reduce cost. Most recipients of awards are hospitals, insurance companies, states, nursing homes, and some community groups. Such projects are localized experiments that, if successful, can be broadened to impact larger groups of patients, and perhaps alter Medicare itself. Accountable Care Organizations (ACOs) are one result of the CMMI's efforts. But as with much the CMMI is doing, the actual utility of ACOs is unknown and, at least to many primary care doctors, just another buden placed on our laps without being contructed with the input of practicing physicians and without having any proven benefit.

While experimentation is both necessary and laudable, it is unclear if the primary recepients of CMMI's dollars are simply more beurocratic agencies that are out of touch with the realities of Medicare and geriatric medicine. Certainly, as with much of the current reform thrust, primary care input is either lacking or absent. Also, without making more fundamental changes in the structure of Medicare, all such efforts are merely band-aides that will be slapped upon a dysfunctional system, thereby assuring their inability to usher in meaningful change. Rather than simply financing pockets of innovation, perhaps the government should talk to those of us who see patients every day and determine which broad changes will be most effective. From there, then real experimentation can begin.

**Total Payment Revenue Budget Cap:** A novel and potentially exciting plan that is gaining a foothold in my state of Maryland involves having the government pay hospitals a global monetary budget every year to provide all health care services. Under such a system hospitals will be more profitable if they can reduce their hospital costs, cut down admissions, and maintain a healthy patient population. Presumably hospitals would work with community doctors and nursing homes to keep patients out of the hospital by treating them at home. If they provide global care cheaper than their historical revenue norms, they profit. If not, they may lose money. Some worry that such a plan will induce hospitals to turn away patients who need hospitalization and to curtail important services. Others believe that hospitals will have no control over admissions and may be put in a precarious financial position.[411]

Ideally, a capitated hospital will be the perfect engine to drive a palliative home care model. Bypassing Medicare, hospitals can pay long-term care facilities and home health agencies directly to keep people out of the hospital, no longer having to adhere to the three-day rule. They can pay for short subacute stays, IV treatments, physical therapy, even custodial care; such payments would save them money if they could keep people out of the hospital. But they may still be hampered by long-term care regulations, by legal liability, and by fear of fraud. It is very unclear if Medicare would even allow such an arrangement to exist. And ultimately hospitals, which would have total control over the entire process, may resort to business as usual, finding other ways to cut cost.

In reality, the most haunting fear that some of us have about such a plan is the centrality of the hospital in scripting it. Likely hospitals will attempt to maximize their own profits by deflecting costs elsewhere in the system, perhaps to outpatient sites that they will own, perhaps to other facilities that perform similar roles such as subacute centers, perhaps to doctors who will have to care for sicker patients without appropriate resources. While this may in itself spur creative ways to care for patients outside the dangerous and expensive hospital walls, it may also simply shift care to other locations no less dangerous and much less sustainable. Also, it must be realized that under current Medicare rules, patients make their own decisions as to whether they choose to utilize the hospital for care, and unless they are incented to stay out of the hospital, there is no advantage for patients to cooperate with the hospitals' goals. Doctors, too, have no incentive to be part of such a plan unless the hospitals buy their practices and make them salaried employees, something that likely will accentuate under this model, or unless somehow doctors are paid and given adequate resources to keep patients out of the hospital. In fact, the end result may be that hospitals will control such a large portion of the entire health care delivery landscape that it is up to them whether successful Medicare reform can be enacted. Whether that is a good recipe for better geriatric care at lower cost has yet to be determined; hospitals do not have a good track record of providing sensible geriatric care. But the capitation may be enough of an incentive to nudge them in the right direction.

## Trying a Different Approach

My experiences with patient care, and ongoing consultation with very experienced colleagues, have led me down a different road than the one current reform efforts are sending us. While I laud both CMS and the ACA for working to fix a very difficult problem, and even for implementing many novel and potentially beneficial solutions, I cannot imagine that these reforms will be successful without a central role for primary care doctors and without a more profound alteration of the current payment system. Thus I propose another way forward.

The crux of my reform ideas center on the basic premise of this book: that aggressive care is not good for older patients, but that Medicare and other players in our health care delivery network are pushing reluctant patients down that dangerous and expensive path. My script does not assume that incentivizing or punishing doctors and hospitals and even drug companies will fix the system. And rather than institute an HMO style of care that shackles patients with unpopular restrictions, true Medicare reform should incentivize patients to pursue sensible and less expensive options. The vast majority of our elderly want to be treated at home and do not seek aggressive care when it is futile. Our current system, even with the proposed reforms that are being implemented, encourages patients to pursue care that most of them do not actually want. The goal of reform, then, is to provide an alternative that is medically sound and that is less expensive for the patient while saving the system needed money.

## The Universal Requirements of Any Reform Effort

From my experience, and from what I have illustrated in this book, I believe that there are certain absolutes that all health care reform must embody. These include:

1.  **Be Cognizant of Americans' disdain for rationed care.** Any reform needs to accept that Americans will not endorse changes that are perceived as rationing. Many years of reform efforts should have taught us that we as a nation are not willing to have administrators and politicians tell us who we can see and what care is appropriate for us or our loved ones. If we simply tell Americans that they can no longer have what they want when they want it, both conservatives and liberals will assault that concept from unique angles, and Americans will reject it entirely.

2.  **Decentralize the Role of Hospitals and Specialists in any Reform Effort.** When the AMA agreed to finally accept Medicare in 1965, it did so with the stipulation that hospitals would remain central players in the medical delivery system. This has been an albatross that is pulling Medicare into its grave. Over the decades there has been no significant decline in the hospital's centrality, while there has been an augmentation of specialization and high-tech medicine. We must move the nexus of reform away from specialists and hospitals and into the realm of primary care, which is the most logical and cost-effective means of achieving improved health care outcomes for the elderly and of saving Medicare money. Hospitals should not be leading this effort, because they have no incentive to alter the status quo, and they are the focus of much of the wasteful and injurious spending that is thrust at our frailest Medicare recipients. There must be a vital role for hospitals in any new version of Medicare, since they do have a crucial place in our health care delivery network. But hospitals must change, and the formula for that change must

trickle up from those who actually practice medicine outside the hospital walls.

3. **Tackle the 25 Percent.** If a company is in financial trouble, and it learns that a quarter of its revenue is being used in a way that is completely wasteful, it will target that spending and reduce the waste. That is the case with Medicare. The fact that a quarter of Medicare's budget is squandered on end-of-life care, where herculean efforts and massive spending lead not to lifesaving results but rather to very difficult and arduous deaths, should be an embarrassment to CMS and to the entire American medical system. Clearly we are not spending our money wisely. No organization, public or private, can justify spending a quarter of its entire budget on something that bears no fruit and leads to no gain. Every reform effort needs to focus on that 25 percent, because any improvement in that number will have significantly positive financial repercussions for our Medicare crisis without curtailing necessary and useful care. Also, knowing that so many of our frail elderly actually are harmed by aggressive medical treatment, one has to wonder if intensive end-of-life care itself contributes to premature death. When we then realize that the vast majority of the elderly actually eschew aggressive end-of-life care and typically only fall prey to it because Medicare gives them no other options, one must wonder why such a system is so entrenched. This is the pond where all Medicare reform must dive, for in it swims the solution to much that is dragging Medicare down.

4. **Provide affordable, sensible alternatives to aggressive care.** It is not enough to simply tell our oldest Medicare recipients to avoid overutilizing specialization and hospitalization. If we as a society seek to curtail aggressive medical treatment at the end of life, then we must provide patients with effective, palliative care either in the home or at other facilities that will not be cost prohibitive. In fact, such care should be less expensive for the patient

than is hospitalization. Also, we must acknowledge that frail patients often require custodial care when they are most sick, they may need intravenous fluid or medicine, and they likely will benefit from rehabilitation and social interaction. This can occur in the home, in assisted-living facilities, in novel acute care geriatric centers, or in current subacute units. Innovative and economical palliative and acute care systems can be devised by our free enterprise system to meet these needs as long as Medicare is willing to finance such care in lieu of hospitalization. It is time to build alternatives to aggressive care before we can effectively tear down the dysfunctional system that now exists.

5. **Acknowledge the worth of death with dignity:** In Washington and Oregon the Death with Dignity Acts allow terminal patients to die by their own volition under the veil of comfort. Patients are prescribed a pill called secobarbital, and those who choose to take the pill on their own will die quietly, typically within a half hour. All eligible people are at the end of life, and most who enter this program cite a lack of autonomy, an inability to engage in enjoyable activities, and a loss of dignity as the reasons for wanting to end their lives.[412] These are the very fears that grip so many of my dementia patients. A majority of patients with early dementia tell us that they do not want to be put in a nursing home and that they do not want any extraordinary medical treatment should they no longer be able to communicate or live an autonomous life. Despite those explicit wishes, far too many frail, demented patients do find themselves both in long-term care and in the claws of an excessively thorough medical delivery system at the end of their lives. With so little that Medicare has to offer them, most have no other option. While it is not likely that our society is ready to allow demented patients to kill themselves, especially when their own judgment is clouded by their disease, such patients, especially when of sound mind, should be given the option to create much more detailed living wills that

stipulate their demands to stay out of the hospital, to be treated only for illnesses that cause discomfort, and to be kept away from medicines and number chasing perceived to prolong life if they so choose. And most significantly, once that document is drafted, it is imperative that it be respected and adhered to. This will allow such patients to live and die with dignity while their dementia erases their minds and decimates their bodies. I refer all readers to *The Best Care Possible* by Ira Byock[413] in which the dying process and the benefits of comfort and dignity during end of life are explored. Too often our patients are muted when they so desperately ask to be left alone and treated with dignity. This must change.

## What Must Happen Before We Instigate Medicare Reform

Medicare certainly plays a large, if unintentional, role in pushing our older patients down a path that is expensive, ineffective, and bereft of compassion. But it is not the only factor involved in twisting our geriatric health care delivery system into something dysfunctional. If we simply repair Medicare, we will be left with other pervasive problems that will need to be surmounted. We should identify and repair those issues first before we attempt to cure Medicare.

**Malpractice Reform.** As long as doctors have a feasible excuse to practice aggressive medicine, they have no incentive to change their habits. And as long as doctors can be successfully sued for practicing sensible medicine, then those who take a less aggressive path risk the blade of litigation. Any changes we make in Medicare must be predicated on the knowledge that in the elderly, less is more. And if such an approach risks malpractice repercussions, then it has no chance of success.

We must dramatically restructure our malpractice system, eliminate pain and suffering rewards, put lawyers at risk for prosecuting questionable cases, and assure that "expert" physicians are scrutinized by the medical community and are subject to significant reprimand if they do make bogus claims. Physicians who are subjected to frivolous suits, something a jury can decide, should be able to be paid by the prosecuting lawyer for the time and income lost during the trial period. Place risk on the lawyers and experts, cut the potential monetary rewards, and the number of suits will diminish. That is just common sense.

**Regulatory Reform:** A recent HHS report estimates that a third of nursing home residents suffer harm due to medical issues that are not discovered by regulators. The report states that over half of serious incidents can be preventable with more regulations, something CMS plans to institute through the ACA this year. An article that describes these efforts suggests that future inspections will now focus on a larger number of medical problems among the frail institutionalized elderly in an effort to prevent problems before they escalate and trigger hospitalizations.[414] But more detailed inspections that put medical problems under a microscope, and that stress thorough monitoring and treatment, will only exacerbate the medicalization and specialization of long term care, leading, as we have shown, to more aggressive care, more hospitalization, and worse outcomes at higher cost. How long will it take for health care reformers to realize that punitive regulations focusing on the attainment of idealized medical outcomes will accomplish the very opposite of what Medicare and our frail elderly want and need?

It is time to erase every nursing home regulation on the books and start from scratch. AMDA would be an ideal shepherd for such change, working with forward thinking facility directors. No longer should facilities be judged by how well they control blood pressure and diabetes, how many residents fall, how many urinary tract infections occur, and how many medicines residents are taking. Rather, nursing homes and assisted-living facilities should be judged by how well they keep residents out of the hospital, how high their retention rate is of nurses and aides, what their nursing aid to resident ratio is, how many of their residents have living wills, and how successful the facility is in providing basic medical care such as immunizations. Also, facilities can be rated on their dementia programs, fall prevention programs, and medicine reduction programs. Nursing homes can be penalized for not properly filling out forms, for procedures that may impair resident safety, and for incidents that may put residents in peril, but these transgressions need to be assessed sensibly on an individual basis and not lead to harsh punishments on first offenses.

Overall the regulatory default button needs to be set on keeping long-term care residents away from tests and aggressive care and out of the hospital. Patients and families who want otherwise will be required to specifically establish orders to make that happen. Sewn into the new regulations must be a realization that the residents of long-term care are frail and sick, are likely to have bad outcomes that are not necessarily anyone's fault, and could be potentially harmed by aggressive care, tight control of their numbers, and hospitalization. The regulations should be simple, should truly reflect quality, and should protect residents from real harm while attempting to encourage facilities to practice innovative and palliative geriatric care.

**Increase the Number of Primary Care Doctors.** No reform effort can survive with a primary care shortage and a specialization glut. We need to incentivize medical students to enter primary care fields, create some degree of salary parity between the various medical fields, and restrict the number of specialty slots available. Given that the free market does not impact physicians' salary, an effort to make physician remuneration fair and more equitable must flow from the insurance company itself, which in our case is Medicare. Such salary alterations can be used to persuade doctors to enter and remain in primary care. As a first step, scripting the salaries of doctors must be removed from the hands of the AMA. An appointed or elected group of physicians affiliated with CMS can work to develop some degree of parity in salary, and at least half of that group should be composed of primary care physicians. With such alterations, the financial windfall inherent to procedure-oriented specialization should be specifically targeted, for as long as more procedures equate to higher income, then not only will there be few students entering primary care, but the entire specialized culture of health care delivery cannot change. It is also imperative that specialty training slots be curtailed, so that we only train the number of specialists we need, rather than the abundance that we are producing now. All of this can be accomplished very easily and without causing significant disruption to the current medical delivery system.

Medical school debt is another contributor to career choice. Graduating with $200,000 debt does not permit most medical students the luxury of following a path of primary care. Some researchers have contemplated cutting medical school by a year in an effort to save money without sacrificing quality. Concluded one study: "there is substantial waste in the education and training of US physicians. Years of training have been added without evidence that they enhance clinical skills or quality of care. This waste adds to the financial burdens of young physicians and increases health care costs."[415]

Interestingly a recent *Washington Post* article about this topic talks about eliminating the fourth year of medical school, which in my opinion is a very crucial year educationally. The article's author interviewed medical school administrators who suggested that any curtailment would necessarily involve the fourth year, with some claiming that a one-year cut "has been tried before, and it was a miserable failure."[416] But in reality, a revamping and trimming of the two preclinical years (the first two years of most medical schools), including moving at least one of those years to becoming part of the undergraduate premed curriculum, would easily allow medicals schools to impart a quality education in three years. With reduction in medical school cost, debt will be a less persuasive factor in career decisions, and this is something that has to be considered more sensibly by reformers. Further, a plan to provide additional debt relief to primary care doctors will push more students in that direction. The government can freeze interest payments and pay off $10,000 of debt a year for students who remain in primary care fields for at least a decade. Such an investment would provide large dividends if it does increase our primary care supply. And without more primary care doctors, Medicare reform cannot succeed.

## Curing Medicare

Fixing Medicare requires financial incentives to convince patients, doctors, and long-term care facilities to pursue less aggressive medical care with a focus on home care and palliative approaches, while incentivizing entrepreneurs to devise creative strategies to provide low-cost quality care for our frail elders. I will outline some specific ideas that my experience has convinced me will be feasible and effective. All of these ideas adhere to the universal reform requirements that I elucidated above. These are but some of many ideas that primary care doctors can provide if only we are involved in Medicare reform.

I do want to emphasize again what I am defining as a palliative approach to care. Palliative care implies that we are more concerned as a health care delivery system with maintaining an elderly patient's dignity, quality of life, and function than we are with extending life. As we have discussed, the "thorough" approach to medical care assumes a central role for medicines, number chasing, tests, procedures, specialization, and hospitalization with the assumption being that the harder we hammer an elderly person with medical aggression, the best chance there is of averting death. Everything we know about geriatrics debunks that myth. In fact, in many conditions, if not all, a palliative approach may lead to a longer life span in addition to its other benefits. My approach, unlike other reform being tossed around, emphasizes the thorough nature of palliative care and the need for Medicare to finance such care, especially when it can be carried out in a patient's own home. Effective palliative care does not, like hospice, assume that a patient is near death. Rather, such a system has as its goal the attainment of happy and productive lives, however long those lives may be.

**The Three-Day Rule Must Die:** Very simply, the existing stipulation that patients must spend three nights in a hospital before receiving payment for subacute care is counterproductive and dangerous. It is also very expensive. Many older people would benefit from rehabilitation and increased care during or after an acute illness, especially care carried out in a nursing home rehabilitation center, a palliative care center, or at home. The fact that they must stay in a hospital to achieve necessary care is complete madness. In the retirement center HMO that I previously discussed we eliminated the three-day rule, and the immediate result was a dramatic reduction of hospitalization. Patients often were admitted directly to the rehabilitation center for acute illness such as pneumonia and dehydration, avoiding the costs and dangers associated with hospitalization. Still others received similar levels of care at home. The HMO paid for those services at a tremendous savings compared to hospitalization and with an immeasurable benefit to our patients. As long as hospitals remain central players in reform efforts, it is unlikely that the three-day rule will disappear, since its elimination will keep countless numbers of elderly patients out of the hospital and thus threaten a large chunk of hospital revenue.

Medicare can and should pay for rehabilitation and home care for very ill patients under physician supervision and with specific goals in mind. The criteria for Medicare payment, and the extent and duration of such payment, can be discussed and delineated. But none of it should be contingent on a prior hospitalization. Once the three-day rule evaporates, then genuine Medicare reform is finally possible.

**Medicare Must Finance Innovation.** With the three-day rule gone, and Medicare now focused on providing effective palliative care out of the hospital, then a crop of innovators will likely fill the gap left by the hospitals' exodus. Once CMS decides what it will pay for, then it can set up demonstration projects whereby entrepreneurial groups can devise novel ways to deliver such care at low cost and high yield. For instance, an agency may be able to provide IV treatments at home, as well as a sufficient number of nurses and aides, bring patients to day-care centers or palliative care centers during the day or when they are too ill for home care, teach families to provide care during nights and weekends, utilize high-tech devices that monitor patients and interact with them, and rent them medical equipment necessary for their particular ailments, potentially for a low price tag. This will be possible once Medicare financing transcends its narrow definition of acute and subacute care. If enterprising Americans know that they will be paid to provide such a service, then they will come to the front lines with some amazing ideas.

The CMS innovation center as it now functions relies too much on a federal top-down approach to reform without altering any of the rules to make effective bottom-up change possible. There is nothing wrong with novel programs funded by the CMS Innovation Center, but to institute meaningful change the bureaucratic hurdles to innovative home-based reform need to be torn down. Until the Medicare playing field is altered, true innovation is not possible. The elderly largely want palliative home care, especially those who understand what that entails. In most instances, they simply cannot afford it, since Medicare will not pay. We already know that such care often is superior. Now it is time to make that our priority and actually finance it. Only then can we persuade our elderly patients to stay out of the hospital, since we will have something better to offer them.

**Offer Nursing Home Eligible Patients a Long-Term Care Bargain.** Most nursing home residents, and their families, prefer to avoid aggressive care and hospitalization. Too often they are pushed in the wrong direction by misguided incentives and disincentives weaved into our current Medicare and regulatory systems. Nursing homes also are rewarded by sending their residents to a hospital when they are ill. With recently enacted reforms under the ACA, hospitalization will be less palatable than treatment within the facility during a very brief thirty-day window after acute hospitalization. Beyond the thirty-day window, though, there are no incentives for the hospital, long-term care facility, or family to avert aggressive care and hospitalization.

Often when a family seeks to avoid aggressive care or hospitalization, they enroll their parents in hospice. While hospice is a wonderful option and does typically keep people out of hospitals, it is very expensive and is often unnecessary. Also under current hospice guidelines, patients can disenroll from hospice, go to the hospital and have it paid for by Medicare, then return back to hospice. In addition, hospice eligibility is becoming more scrutinized, and fewer demented long-term care residents qualify. Finally, hospice assumes that death is imminent, something that many patients and families are not ready to accept. Therefore, hospice is not a viable buffer to aggressive care for everyone, and much of what if offers does not meet the needs of demented long-term care residents who simply want to maintain their comfort and dignity.

Similarly, some families want to keep their demented parent at home but cannot afford home health care, day-care programs, and other necessary support mechanisms to enable them to care for their aging relatives while still being able to live their own lives. Such families often are forced to send their loved ones to nursing homes, where eventually Medicaid picks up the tab after all of their own money evaporates.

There is another option that should be explored, one that would be beneficial to nursing homes, welcomed by patients and families, provide better and more compassionate care to the frail elderly, and save money by averting hospitalization and specialization. Medicare currently pays $12,000 per enrollee per year, on average, for health care costs. Much more than that is spent on the oldest and frailest elderly, some of whom live in nursing homes: money typically being used to cover unnecessary excessive care including hospitalization. While Medicare is happy to pay for hospital stays, emergency room visits, tests, procedures, and specialist visits, the most basic care needed by families—either home care, day care, or nursing home care—must be paid by the families themselves since it is out of Medicare's purview. And when families do run out of money, Medicaid will typically pay only for nursing home care, rarely financing enough home care services to make home care feasible.

I suggest that nursing home residents be offered a better and cheaper option through Medicare. The residents who accept this option—the palliative care option—will agree to forgo most testing, specialist visits, and hospitalization in exchange for Medicare paying a certain amount toward either nursing home care, assisted-living care, or various home care options. Medicare will continue to pay for basic lab tests, x-rays, primary care visits within the facility/home, podiatry visits, and on-site visual/hearing visits. When nursing home residents are ill, Medicare will pay for acute care within the facility or at home. But if residents under the palliative care option want to be hospitalized, or see their cardiologists, or get MRIs for back pain, they will have a deductible to pay before Medicare kicks in, and that deductible will equal or even exceed the amount of money that Medicare will be paying toward their annual long-term care costs. In other words, if Medicare pays $10,000 annually to help defray costs for long-term care and home care patients who sign up for the palliative care option, that $10,000, or even a bit more, will become the deductible such patients will have to pay for well-defined aggressive services such as hospitalization and specialization before Medicare starts paying.

For such a system to work, the payment process must be altered. Currently, nursing home residents who exhaust their finances can apply for a Medicaid waiver. Under the waiver, Medicaid pays the cost of a resident's nursing home bill, and Medicare B pays for all medical costs. Under the new system, the Medicaid waiver will only kick in every year after a resident pays the first $10,000 of his long-term care fee out of pocket, money available to the resident by Medicare if he chooses the palliative care option. In addition, Medicaid must be willing to pay for assisted-living and home care to assure that patients who deplete their funds will not have to be tossed into a much more expensive and often undesirable nursing home if they prefer other options. While the palliative care option will not pay for the entirety of home or long-term care, it will at least help defray costs, and especially with innovative home care options becoming available, it may truly allow older people to stay at home.

Most significantly, under the palliative care option, residents and their families now have a real incentive to do the right thing. Keeping their loved ones out of the hospital and away from specialized and excessive care actually will save them money. Thus they can pursue a medically sound course without being financially penalized. Such a plan does not prevent patients and their families from pursing aggressive care if they so choose; there are no restrictions put in place unless they sign up for the palliative care option. And even if they do sign up and then choose to take a more aggressive route or to hospitalize their loved one, they merely have to repay the $10,000 stipend given to them (since that is their deductible) by CMS before Medicare starts paying for aggressive care again. Choice is not expunged; rather, patients are given more options, and are financially rewarded for keeping their loved ones out of harm's way. To cut back hospitalization in the nursing home eligible population by providing families with alternatives not only will be cost saving for the system, but will also allow Medicare to deliver superior care. Families deserve financial assistance in caring for their loved ones in a manner that is compassionate and effective.

**Reform the Medicare Drug Plan.** Medicare D pays for medications. Unlike reasonable systems, like at the VA and many HMOs, our Medicare D program does not negotiate with pharmaceutical companies to secure the best cost, nor does it allow only generic drugs when applicable. If patients are to receive medication at taxpayer expense, they have to be given cost effective choices for which the government pays less. If patients do not approve of these restrictions, they can easily join secondary insurance plans that will give them what they desire, or simply pay for their medicines out of pocket and not sign up for Medicare D. But there is no reasonable excuse to provide a drug plan and publicly finance it unless it makes economic and medical sense. A pragmatic drug plan will save millions of dollars for Medicare without impacting patient care.

**Allow Physicians to Interact with Patients and Families More Creatively.** I recall that when I first started my practice I received several calls one day from family members of my patients who wanted to talk to me. That afternoon I had to drop off my car at the service station, and while I walked home I decided to call the family members back. When I finally reached my house forty minutes later, the first son was still talking to me, and he had a lot more to say. During the first few months of practice I continued to be burdened by similarly prolonged phone conversations in increasing numbers, while also having families asking to meet with me to discuss their dad or mom. On certain days I would spend several hours answering calls and meeting with families, none of which is reimbursed by Medicare. Medicare prevents me from charging a fee for these services at all unless I see the patient face-to-face on the same day. Finally I realized that I could no longer afford this level of care, and I required all family members to contact me either by email or by attending their parents' visits.

To this day I still receive approximately a hundred emails and messages daily, some of which are long and complicated, all of which require extensive nonreimbursed time and often complex decision making. Although still consuming several hours a day, communicating electronically rather than by phone enables me to converse with patients, families, nurses, therapists, and others and yet is not so onerous that it cuts into my ability to see patients, which is the only theater of my job that Medicare is willing to compensate and for which I am allowed to charge. But phone calls and meetings are very valuable to good geriatric care. Often they enable me to keep people out of the hospital, to redefine care plans, and to discuss with caregivers the many hurdles that are tossed at them. Also, with technology constantly evolving, it is possible that I can call patients and, with telemedicine, essentially conduct home visits remotely. This too is not covered by Medicare, nor can I legally charge patients for this service if I am a Medicare provider.

Another use of electronic medicine that would be very helpful for patient and doctor alike, and that is being used in the VA system, is remote consultation. Often we would like the advice of a specialist but do not feel that our patient needs to be followed by or even to see that specialist. Through telemedicine we could have access to specialty consultation during an office visit, something that an enterprising company could easily make happen if it were paid for such consultations. Again, although it may cost Medicare some money up front, this form of consultation will cut down on specialty care and put more control in the hands of primary care doctors who can more intelligently utilize specialty services. Patients too would benefit, as they would not have to make multiple trips to doctors, while Medicare would likely pay much less for remote consultation than it would for an office visit.

It is time that Medicare allows physicians some freedom to establish programs that are cost effective and medially sensible and that transcend the narrow window of what Medicare will currently finance. Likely some of these programs will not be covered by Medicare, such as phone calls, but at least Medicare should allow physicians to charge their patients a fee for providing an important and time-consuming service. Phone calls, telemedicine, family meetings, remote consultation, and other creative means of interaction take time and help enhance the care of our older patients even if they do not involve direct patient contact and a medically oriented script. Such strategies will help patients and families negotiate the many perils of aging without having to schedule visits that are logistically difficult and typically dominated by strict health care issues and by us having to concentrate on completing our scripted notes. And it will save Medicare money by allowing us to work with families and keep patients away from aggressive care, as well as permitting us to evaluate and treat patients who are too frail to get to our office. Medicare would be wise to loosen its grip on our ability to take care of our patients and to innovate.

**Enact a System of Copays:** Establishing copays for services will enable CMS to steer patients in certain directions within the health care continuum without having to enact painful rationing. Copays are sensible parts of many medical insurance plans, but they do not exist in Medicare. Under current law, Medicare B patients have to pay 20 percent of all their care, and such an expense certainly could impact behavior if a patient does not also carry secondary insurance that typically pays the remaining cost of care. But the vast majority of patients do carry secondary insurance, and thus the current system does not dissuade them from leaping upon the wagon of thorough and getting all the tests, procedures, and specialist visits they want, or that they are told they need, without paying anything out of their pockets. In other words, patients have no financial stake in the system that might give them pause when they are told they need a certain test or procedure. The situation is even more telling with Medicare A and hospitalization when, after a deductible that is typically paid by secondary insurance, patients get virtually all services fully funded by Medicare. As we have discussed, because of the everything-is-free Medicare payment structure, it is less expensive for patients to be hospitalized than to try to negotiate a more sensible course of medical care at home.

What will copays accomplish? Copays would not be covered by secondary insurances and would vary based on the particular type of medical service being offered. For every visit, test, procedure, or hospitalization, patients would be asked to pay a specified amount of money on top of what insurance pays. Those services that are more costly and less efficacious would require higher copays. With an out-of-pocket payment staring them in the face for a certain procedure, such as an MRI for back pain, a patient may then pause and ask if such services are necessary. Copays, then, by giving patients some financial risk in their decisions, could be designed to pull patients down a more prudent and less expensive path of care. Patients will retain their ability to choose which path they pursue, and can be as "thorough" as they wish without restriction, but they may find that the less aggressive paths are more appealing if they incur smaller copays.

Under a copay system, patients would no longer pay a deductible. Instead, they would pay copays throughout the year every time they use a certain service. For patients who barely utilize the health care system, such a scenario would save them money since their total copay allocation would likely be less than the cost of their deductible. For excessive users, the out-of-pocket costs would escalate the more services they utilize. Of course, Medicare would still pay for the majority of health care, but the small copays would defer some of Medicare's payment to the patient, thus giving patients just enough skin in the game to force them to contemplate the utility of their decisions.

Copays will be designed to open some paths and clutter others. For example, visits to primary care doctors will require no copay. Medicare will pay its traditional 80 percent and secondary insurance will pay the other 20 percent, but patients will not have to pay anything up front. This will encourage patients to see their primary care physicians first before taking other paths. Similarly, certain tests and procedures will incur no copays, including immunization, appropriate screening, basic blood tests, and even rehabilitation and some home care. The goal is to encourage patients to seek out effective forms of care and prevention without incurring any additional cost.

Most other services will require patients to pay a copay up front, and this is money that neither Medicare nor secondary insurance will pay. It is also money that doctors/facilities will need to collect from patients, as insurance will pay them a reimbursement that is reduced by the amount of the copay. For instance, if a visit or procedure costs $200, then under the old system Medicare pays the physician or facility $160 (80 percent) and the patient's secondary insurance pays the other $40 (20 percent). Under the new system, if there is a $50 copay, then the doctor/facility will collect $50 from the patient at the time of the visit. Medicare will then pay the physician $120 and the patient's secondary will pay $30. The physician/facility will earn the same amount of money, but more of it will come directly from the patient and less from Medicare. In fact, in the scenario I illustrated, Medicare would pay $40 less per visit, and thus CMS would save money immediately without having to reduce physician or procedure reimbursement. Also, since the amount that the secondary insurance company will be required to pay will be reduced, it is very conceivable that the cost of secondary policies will decrease. But most importantly, such a system, if smartly designed, will reward patients who utilize services with smaller copays rather than those with higher copays such as specialty visits, expensive tests, procedures, and hospitalization.

Visits to specialists may incur a $50 copay. If a patient needs to see a specialist, then that cost will not be prohibitive, unless the patient wants to see specialists frequently. The fact is that primary care physicians are trained to handle the vast majority of medical problems, and the copay system would put the crux of care again in their hands. Certain specialty visits may be exempt from copays including annual ophthalmologic visits, specified visits for post-operative care, or oncologic visits for patients actively receiving chemotherapy. Patients can continue to see all their specialists as often as they would like, but would have to pay for such a service.

Procedures will also be subject to copays. MRIs may cost the patient $100 up front, which is $100 less that Medicare has to pay. Again, this will force patients to contemplate whether that spine MRI or repeat echocardiogram is really necessary. Stress tests, ultrasounds, CT scans, etc., will all be subject to copays of various amounts. None of those copays will be so onerous as to prevent any patient from obtaining a necessary test, but the extra cost will give patients some pause.

Hospitals and emergency rooms will also charge a copay. Again, for the few times patients need to go to a hospital, these copays will not prevent them from obtaining necessary services; most car repairs cost more. But charging patients a global fee of $200 for every emergency room visit, and another $200 for subsequent hospital admission, will force patients and doctors to really make sure that hospitalization is necessary, especially since the three-day rule has been eliminated and other less expensive options for care will exist.

One goal of copays is to encourage patients to be treated at home. Currently home care is expensive and can only provide limited services, but that can easily be changed, especially if home health copays are less than those charged in the hospital.

Home IV therapy, home antibiotics, home health aides, home health nursing, home health rehabilitation, and home palliative services: all of these options should not only be offered by Medicare, but they should be far less expensive to the patient than should the option of hospitalization. Medicare can pay for a certain amount of home health aides, physical therapy, nursing, treatment, and monitoring, all with nominal copays. If a sick patient cannot be treated at home, because he is unable to find family or friends to help him through the tough times when aides are not available, or he needs more help than an aide can provide, then Medicare should pay him to get treatment in a subacute facility or palliative care center. The copay for such service should also be significantly less than a hospital copay. These facilities have twenty-four-hour nursing care; ample aides to take care of basic needs; access to intravenous fluids and medicines; appropriate medical equipment, oxygen, nebulizers, and blood testing; and primary care doctors and geriatric nurse practitioners who will visit, all provided at a fraction of the cost as would be incurred in a hospital. Also, long-term care facilities are safer than hospitals in regard to infection and iatrogensis, have no specialists or expensive tests on-site, and will be less inclined to launch their residents into the morass of aggressive medical care when their patients will have to pay a large copay if they are sent to the hospital.

Many reformers worry about home health care abuse, and they have good reason for this concern. Home health fraud is rampant, and it costs Medicare millions of dollars every year. But appropriate home health care is humane and cost saving. The price tag would pale in comparison to hospitalization, and the safety and dignity would be far superior. Home care needs to be a viable option if Medicare is going to shed its current obsession with aggressive care. As is the case with all agencies that obtain money from the government, fraud needs to be extirpated, but the fear of fraud should not deter Medicare from paying for the most appropriate and cost-saving services.

Creative copays will be necessary for various conditions. What will be done about dialysis, chemotherapy, and drug injections that are given regularly? In my opinion, dialysis will incur an annual copay as well as a monthly Medicare payment to the dialysis center; if dialysis centers and renal doctors can determine a means of reducing the number of times someone has to be dialyzed in a month, then they will earn more money since they are paid a global amount every month. Similar systems can be set up for surgeries, chemotherapy, radiation treatment, specialized injections such as remicaid. In those cases, there can be a global payment and copay for the entirety of the procedure/treatment.

The expectation is that copays would be collected directly by the providing doctor or facility up front. Copays can be negotiated. While CMS will set the copay upper limit, doctors or facilities will have the authority to reduce the amount charged due to special circumstances, such as the inability for a patient to pay, or as an attempt to reduce cost to patients and thus gain a competitive advantage over other doctors or facilities. The latter is perhaps best illustrated by considering a radiology facility. One facility may purchase all of the newest and most flashy MRI and CT scanners and advertise that they have the latest in technology. Another facility may rely on older but still excellent machines, and instead advertise that they will waive or reduce the copay. Similarly, a cardiologist who has to see a patient several times a year for a pacemaker check, something that constitutes a brief and simple visit, may elect to waive the copay for that service, thus attracting more such patients into his practice. Capitalism in the health care field is nonexistent at present, since all rates are predetermined, but with copays modest competition for pricing can occur, at least at a low level.

The precise amount of copays to be charged will be determined by CMS. The goal is to elevate charges for inefficient and overutilized parts of our health care delivery system and reduce the cost for visits and treatments whose use is to be encouraged. The result is fivefold. First, patients still have a full choice of which doctors, tests, and procedures they will use; no committee or set of rules will infringe upon that right, and there will be no rationing of care. Second, since patients will be expected to pay at least some of most charges, Medicare will be paying less, and this alone will save it millions of dollars every year. Third, patients will be reluctant to pursue a course that is more expensive unless they

are given good reason to do so. Thus patients can steer themselves down
a more sensible and cost-effective course through financial incentives
and disincentives. Fourth, primary care doctors will gain some financial
advantage in the system since they will not have to charge copays and
thus will receive more secure reimbursement. While some parity in payment between specialists and primary care doctors must be a part of
any reform model, the copay system offers primary care a small leap in
status without CMS having to cut specialist pay. Fifth, a copay model will
spark innovation in health care delivery, especially with regards to palliative and home care, since home care services will be less expensive to
patients due to lower copays.

Copays are a facile, flexible, and fair means of nudging patients
down a better path. No choice will be restricted. Thorough care will not
be denied, although it may become more expensive than more sensible
alternatives. There is no political reason to buck copays, physicians will
not have their incomes altered, and the basic fee-for-service payment
system will remain intact. It is in fact a very simple method to achieve
dramatic change.

**Unify Medicare into a Single Insurance Plan.** Once all of the above
reforms are enacted, none of which will require a major restructur-
ing of Medicare, then a more substantial change could be completed.
Currently Medicare is divided into A, B, and D. There are good reasons
for this split. It is felt that those people who cannot afford to pay for
Medicare B should at least have access to a hospital level of care should
something dramatic, such as a burst appendix, require them to have an
expensive intervention. This is considered catastrophic insurance. Every
elderly American thus is given Medicare A, while only those Americans
who want outpatient insurance will pay Medicare B premiums. But as we
have seen, that demarcation has eroded over time. The vast majority of
Americans, well over 90 percent, have both Medicare B and a secondary insurance. In fact, the total annual cost for Medicare B premiums
and the deductible is $1405.80,[417] a cost that elderly Americans can typi-
cally afford and that makes good financial sense. By having Medicare

A separate and playing by different rules, a very confusing system has been enacted: one that, as we have seen, can lead to dysfunctional and expensive health care provision.

A unified system that eliminates the letters A-D and gives all Americans Medicare coverage will be far simpler. Any such system would need to be cognizant of the need to still provide catastrophic insurance for those unable to pay, and will have to also accept that hospitalization, which is often necessary and very expensive, must have its costs capped. Under such a system people can have four choices: Medicare with high copays, Medicare with lower copays, and both of those with or without drug coverage. The high copay option would cost people less money up front (perhaps $500/year) but would incur higher copays for each service. The low copay option would cost more per year (probably the $1500 that is now being paid for Medicare B), but would cost less in co-pays. Under both systems the hospital copays would remain very high. Also, in both scenarios, Medicare would pay 80 percent of all services up to a certain defined cap, after which it will pay 100 percent, thus allowing patients with expensive hospital stays or special needs such as chemotherapy to be able to afford such services even if they do not have secondary insurance. Copays would of course continue to apply even if Medicare is paying 100 percent of cost. The high copay system will appeal to younger and healthier Medicare patients, while the lower copay system will be more sensible for those who are sicker.

As with all reforms I have tossed about in this chapter, it is important to field test the concepts and calculate cost before implementing any comprehensive program. These are ideas that derive from my primary care experience and that I believe would do much to alleviate our financial and health care crises in this country. I am no economist or policy expert. But I am a doctor, and Medicare has been with me from the start. I know what works and what does not. And certainly for any real change to occur we must surmount the political and societal hurdles that are piled in our path, redefine thorough care, and engineer real changes that can allow us to care for our elderly patients properly.

And that is it. Simple and direct. The goal is an easy one. Let Medicare be a sustainable tool to enable Americans to age in a stress-free, secure, and dignified manner. Medicare no longer need be that monstrous albatross that is expanding our budget deficit and destroying our economy in its quest to do all things for all people. Rather it should be sensible and reasonable, seeking to encourage medical care that is known to be effective in the elderly rather than care that is wasteful and potentially dangerous. After a little nudging, some innovation, and a few rule changes, Medicare will thus be a fully affordable insurance that will care for us and our children for many decades to come.

Society has defined thorough care as a search for perpetual life by overtreating, overtesting, and engaging on a quixotic quest for the un-achievable through specialization and hospitalization. We know that such a definition of thorough is actually backward, and that aggressive care causes harm at great financial and physical cost. Medicare can be the instrument to help us obtain better care for our elders, not the high-cost specialized care that it is financing currently. To those who seek more than Medicare will deliver, then their pocketbooks can be open as wide as they so desire to pay copays and long-term care bills. But to those who seek to age gracefully, Medicare will be there in perpetuity to guide us along the way.

# AFTERWORD

## REDEFINING THOROUGH

*"Our society must make it right and possible for old people
not to fear the young or be deserted by them, for the test of a
civilization is the way it cares for its helpless members."*
*Pearl Buck, Nobel Prize winning novelist*

Today I saw a patient who looked great. Almost eighty, in a retirement community, Mrs. W. had come to a certain peace in her life. She had been very anxious, struggling with pain everywhere, worsening balance, high blood pressure and high sugar, fatigue, and depression. She saw doctors and specialists with great regularity, flooded her body with medicines and tests, and was always looking for a fix. She could not leave her apartment, and was losing weight. Now all that had improved and she glowed.

"I am fighting the good fight," she told me. "And I am winning."

The good fight had changed its focus over the past few months for Mrs. W. Until recently she attempted through various devices and doctor visits to eliminate her pain, to fix her balance and find out why she was so shaky, to worry about her blood pressure and sugars that she checked incessantly, to wonder what had become of her that now she had been forced to exist in a retirement community with so many old people. But at some point an epiphany overcame her thoughts. Now the good fight meant that she was going to persevere despite all of the problems that gnawed at her. She stopped all but a couple of pills, and her sugars and pressure actually improved. She walked with a walker and had become more social; now she taught a class on spirituality in her retirement community, helping others to come to peace with themselves.

"I no longer ask why," she told me. "I just move on and do what I can. And I am trying to help others do the same. By helping them, I'm helping myself."

Mrs. W. had come to a point in her life where she stopped trying to cure her aging. She in fact started to redefine thorough. She no longer adhered to the accepted dogma that with aggressive posturing she could defeat the many ailments and diseases that struck her. She did not chase numbers, ask for more tests, put herself on countless medicines, and seek specialty care. Rather she accommodated to aging and she thrived. To her, thorough no longer implied being tested and treated to death in an effort to achieve something that continued to frustrate and elude her. Now thorough meant to work hard in all facets of her life so that she could live and thrive despite her aliments. Thorough was not something that a doctor or test or drug was going to give to her. Thorough was the mental and physical discipline that was now her responsibility so she could become a healthier and happier person.

Despite all we do not know about medical treatment of the elderly, especially those with memory loss and dementia, we do know that an active lifestyle that emphasizes socialization and exercise can achieve successful improvement in symptoms and quality of life.[418] [419] [420] [421] In my experience, those who look past their ailments and live their lives to the fullest are the ones who age the most successfully and who are the happiest.

One of my favorite patients, 93 year old Mr. P., was a tiny Italian man who typically came in with his pleasant son for our every-three-month visits. He had a litany of medical problems, most of which were either quiet or of no concern to him, and overall he remained active and healthy, without much to relay to me; he accepted and accommodated to aging very well. His son too did not want to look for problems, and often we talked about issues of the day, or other more mundane topics such as the soups they were serving at his retirement community. His son took him on trips frequently, and even became a shuttle driver at the community where his father lived so he could see his father more and help others in his father's shoes.

One day I saw that Mr. P. made an acute visit to see me, and I asked my front staff why he was coming in.

"He wouldn't tell us," the receptionist said to me. "But he said it was urgent that he see you today."

I feared that this man who complained about nothing must have a catastrophic illness; why else would he demand to see me today? But when he arrived in the office, he looked great.

"Hey doc," he said with his typical smile. "I've got heart disease, diabetes, high blood pressure, I pee too much from a big prostate, and my balance isn't worth a damn. You can write all that stuff in your note and bill Medicare for it and say we talked about it. But let me tell you why I am really here."

I peered at him inquisitively.

"I'm taking a Jewish history class at the community college, which is a great class, but there's a lot of confusing things they talk about for a Catholic like me, and I know you're Jewish, and you like history, so I was wondering if I could run some stuff by you."

That was the urgent visit! And both of us enjoyed it very much.

But after discussing a bit of history, we did talk about him, how he was feeling, what his expectations were for the rest of his life, his exercise regime, his family. I learned more about Mr. P. during that visit than I had in all my previous medical encounters. Never did I put a blood pressure cuff on his arm, whip out my stethoscope, or suggest checking labs. I did not even dance my hands across the computer keyboard desperately scripting Medicare's requisite note. I merely followed his agenda. For a brief moment I stepped outside the narrow cage into which society and Medicare has shoved me as I care for my patients. Instead I became Mr. P.'s doctor.

Looking back on Mr. P's visit and others that have been similar, I realize that we are defining thorough all wrong. To be a thorough doctor is not only about ordering tests and prescribing medicines and checking numbers that we can fix. That is an easy way to satisfy everyone and accomplish nothing. To be really thorough is to hold back from being aggressive. To explain to my patients why certain labs and treatments are not appropriate despite what they may have read in the *Washington Post* or heard from their neighbor. To have the guts not to listen to their heart with my stethoscope or check their blood pressure. To be thorough is to talk to them about their lives, their futures, their fears, and their limitations and to help them surmount the ravages of aging. That discussion may not always involve an exam or even a medical vocabulary. But it is the most thorough way that we as doctors can interact with and succor our elderly patients.

Being thorough is very difficult, because the script tells us and our patients that we are supposed to be checking and looking and measuring. Medicare's formulaic template notes that doctors must complete at every visit to be compliant with their rules insist that we assess a specified number of complaints, record a specified amount of measurements, examine a specified amount of their body, and review a specified number of problems. Even Medicare's wellness visit, which was a gift to primary care from CMS because it allows us to spend time with our patients once a year without having to delve into their medical problems, is built with a preordained template of clinical practice guidelines that we must complete exactly as Medicare states. Unfortunately, that template often does not jibe with my elderly patients' lives or needs, and its questions have no meaning for those who live in long-term care or are too confused to respond. Medicare, and the society that fuels it, has defined thorough as being aggressive, and that philosophy is imprinted on every action we are required to take. But that is not what the elderly need. And that approach is expensive and ineffective, even if it is the simplest path to take. We as a society, and we as a medical community, must redefine thorough. That is what will cure Medicare.

The public perception of my profession is a dreary one. Caring for the elderly engenders images of decay, decline, mental collapse, gas, wet diapers, walkers, electric carts, hearing aids, and of course the siren of an ambulance taking yet another old guy to the hospital. All of these images are, of course, correct, and on any given day I am confronted with each of these situations, and I also fill out any number of death certificates, saying goodbye to another of my patients, a victim of the inevitability of aging.

But my job is so much more than that. Its concealed beauty reminds me of my four years of medical school in the North Bronx. When people visited me there they pointed out the congestion, graffiti, and garbage in the street. But being there I became numb to all of that. Instead I enjoyed the wonderful food, smells, vitality, and landscape; the best running trails I ever darted upon traversed the wilderness of the Bronx. And when I view my job now, I am numb to the overt signs of aging that my patients wear every day. Rather I see only beauty. Within each of my patients is a full life that has been lived, a vitality that sadly is often stripped away in their feckless fight to defeat age. Within each of my patients is a story and an enduring spark and that is what I seek to discover and ferment, rather than merely being a robotic technician who fixes numbers and pushes the false allure of thorough.

The heart and soul of my job emanates from the patients for whom I have the honor to care and who are so much deeper than the diagnoses and numbers that have come to define them. I have met patients who worked with famous politicians and scientists, and some who shared some quiet fame on their own. I have lived through D-day and Okinawa, have been aboard ships at Midway where explosions caused asbestos snow storms and the entire crew shit in their pants. I have lived the life of POWs in Germany trading cigarettes for food, and of men on the front line watching as their friends were picked off one by one. Just the other day I met a new patient in his nineties who was on the airfields of Pearl Harbor when it was attacked, and he felt that every Japanese plane that dived down was trying to kill him personally. I have taken care of

German women who lived through the bombing of Berlin and witnessed the deaths of most of their family members, and Jews who survived the gas chambers. Even the most demented of the veterans and war victims I have come to know, the ones who no longer recognize their wife and kids and don't know a spoon from a pen, can recall their military units and battles with clarity and emotion. From teachers, to salesmen, to victims of racist attacks, to artists and astronauts, my patients are the very embodiments of living history. They relish telling their stories, and in many ways those stories encapsulate who they are and define how they think.

Sadly, only after many of my patients die do I get to know them. I remember one demented man from the nursing home who often climbed into women's beds and who spit on the nursing aides. To us, he was quite pathetic. When he died, no one thought much about it. Two days later I picked up a copy of the *Baltimore Sun* and stumbled upon a quarter page obituary near a picture of a young man smiling brightly holding a trumpet and surrounded by cheering soldiers. It turns out that this man had been instrumental in founding the USO, and then had gone on to be a successful corporate leader who helped modernize the army's supply network. To many people quoted in the obituary, the man was a hero. It saddened me that I had not known that before. I cared more about his blood pressure, his medicines, and his behavior than who he actually was. Perhaps I could have sparked some of those memories and helped the man get through what must have been the most painful and demeaning part of his incredible life.

Throughout my many years of practicing geriatric medicine, I am most amazed by those patients and families who can look beyond their problems, who can transcend the overwhelming dogma pounded into our brains that more is better and that answers and solutions for everything exist if we try hard enough, and who come to peace with their aging process and learn to live with it by accommodating and persevering. If this book is designed to show anything it is that successful aging need not be burdened by the constant struggle to defeat the inevitable. That fight very often leads to disastrous consequences, at a very high cost to the patients and to society. Successful aging is so much more rewarding, and that is what I try so hard to promote at every turn. Unfortunately my message that the elderly can best help themselves through physical and mental discipline is often trumped by the false allure of hope ingrained in the seed of thorough, a message trumpeted by pharmaceutical companies, the lay press, specialization, our medical leaders, and Medicare itself that there is an answer out there for everything if you just keep poking yourself enough, taking enough medicines, and rushing to the hospital when you get too sick. That is my most daunting enemy, and it is a lethal weed that is choking Medicare's hope for survival.

It is difficult for most patients and families to view health care under the lens of common sense. Not when we live in a society that thrives on excess. There is always a story of someone saved by a procedure or test who is just like mom. Always a glimmer of hope hanging just beyond our reach. Always someone who thinks there is an answer to every problem, or at least there should be. Always a doctor willing to be the hero.

So therefore, it is up to us to redefine thorough and help our patients live better than the dogma allows. I view myself as a guide through the older years, an individual who can help my patients understand, accept, and adjust to the many hazards that barrage us as we age. I try to teach my patients, and their families, to continue living and thriving despite the tide of illness and disability thrust at them. Rather than medicate people, I try to withdraw medicine. Rather than searching for disease, I try to avoid looking too hard. Rather than aggressively treating ailments such as diabetes and high blood pressure, I try to convince my elderly patients to back off and not worry. To me, the enemies of successful aging are stress and inactivity, and very often the quest for immortality through medical thoroughness only accelerates both of these demons. I try to retreat from hard-core medical dogma scripted by experts in the form of clinical guidelines, and instead learn to concoct individualized strategies to help my patients maintain their vitality. Sometimes it is difficult for old people and their kids to accept this minimalistic outlook.

But medical studies have proven its wisdom, and those of us in the field treat it like gospel based on our ample experience.

Every elderly person lives within a delicate balance between function and disease. Even those who look good externally are standing one insult away from a cascade that may unravel everything. A good doctor knows that. A good doctor is not one who looks for problems, who seeks perfection in numbers, who adds stress to their patients' lives by tossing tests and specialists at them, and who is oblivious to the precarious balance within their patients' bodies. A good doctor is one who knows you well, who holds your hand, and who helps guide you through the medical theater in which you are enjoying the final act. A good doctor has the guts to put on the breaks. When we back off, almost everything improves. Backing off is not giving up. It is the best medicine we have. It is akin to hope. It is truly thorough care.

Medicare does not facilitate successful aging. It does not reward or assist those who take a path of less aggressive care. Often, in fact, it gets in the way. By paying for specialization and hospitalization, for tests and procedures, for the most aggressive of care, it sends patients down a road that is traumatic and stressful. By not paying for most home treatments, for nursing aides and phone calls to a doctor, for palliative long-term care and the ability for families to keep the elderly at home, Medicare turns its back on quality and dignity.

When I titled this book, I initially named it after one of my patient's daughters who jokingly anointed herself as "the Boss." The Boss helped me to understand that the most thorough patient advocate is not necessarily the one who most bombastically demands to dive into the teeth of a health care delivery system that Medicare will gladly finance. Rather, a truly thorough family member, like the Boss, is one who aggressively provides comfort and dignity in someone's final years, and who fights against a system and a society that would have her do otherwise. The Boss was that person, and her thoroughness paid off.

The Boss's mother was my patient for more than a decade. Mrs. Lo was a small, pleasant lady who spoke very slowly and repeated herself often. She saw me for visits every three months, typically to discuss her diabetes, some minor aches and pains, and her many stories from Poland where she was born. Overall Mrs. Lo was very healthy as she entered her nineties, still independent, and not crippled by any serious medical problems. But her mind was slowly deteriorating, and her ability to carry out simple activities of daily living became an increasing burden of which she was never aware but that clearly impacted her life.

I had heard from her daughter sparingly prior to her more pronounced memory loss, but by her mother's late eighties the daughter started to call me often, often tremulous, shooting me a list of Mrs. Lo's most recent sugars, talking about her poor balance, and then asking: "She's going to be OK, right? She's not going to die, right?" The Boss, as she labeled herself due to the fact that she had now put herself in charge of her mom's life, loved her mom as excessively as anyone ever loved anyone else. She could not imagine life without her.

So, unmarried and without kids, she found a night job, and she spent her days with her mom. She took her on trips to restaurants and stores, talked about making an excursion to Poland sometime soon, and more than anything kept her mom happy and mobile and independent.

When I first met the Boss she assaulted me with a threatening proclamation: "I want you to know that I am going to do whatever it takes to keep my mother alive, and I expect you to do the same, doctor." I thought, OK, here's another one of those family members, the ones who treat their parents like little children, drag them from doctor to doctor and test to test, dominate appointments without letting their parents get in a word edgewise, and ultimately drive their parents into an early and painful grave at great financial and personal expense.

But the Boss was not like that.

Yes, she called me a lot, typically with an alarmist charm about her. But never did she demand anything other than reassurance.

"Mom's diabetes is out of control, doctor," she said to me, more than just once, reading me a list of sugars that were not very high. "Should we be changing her medicine? Should I be worried? Should we be taking her to an endocrinologist? My sister says these sugars are going to kill her. She is going to be OK, right?"

"Well, those numbers look good to me, but if you want her to go to an endocrinologist, you don't need my permission. Medicare lets you take her to whomever you want whenever you want to."

"Doctor, I just want to know that we are doing the right thing and she'll be OK."

"I think she's doing great," I told the Boss.

"Really? She will be OK? Thank you, doctor. Thank you."

The calls were brief and predictable, and the when the Boss called I always called her right back. It took just a minute of time, and once I gave the magic word that all was OK she brought her mom on another walk, or trip, or imaginary adventure in Poland.

And so it went. "Does my mom need a mammogram, doctor?"

"Not at ninety-two."

"But she'll be all right, right doctor? She won't die of breast cancer, right?"

"There's probably a higher risk of her getting hit by a car on the way to the test."

"Do you think she'll die of a car accident?"

If I ever suggested a test, or even a specialist appointment as benign as an eye doctor, the Boss bucked. She clearly did not want to put her mother through all of that, even though she asked about it incessantly. Being barraged by a society that believes in excess, the Boss needed constant reassurance from me to do what she knew was right by way of her mother. She needed me to alleviate her stress so she could relieve her mother's. So, from my perspective, everything was OK. Everything would always be OK.

One day the Boss took her mother for a walk in the hall and accidently tripped her mother, who tumbled down and slammed onto her back. Mrs. Lo did not walk again for three months, and the Boss was overcome with guilt. But I continued to deflect the blame (carpets, lighting, poor vision), to help the Boss keep her mom out the a hospital or nursing home (I wrote many letters to her employer to allow her to stay with her mom and arranged some home health, none of which Medicare helped cover), and kept her away from narcotics and specialists and other interventions that might cause her harm. We talked daily on the phone ("She'll be all right, won't she doctor? I didn't kill her did I?"), and I visited her a few times, and eventually Mrs. Lo resumed her car rides and her walks and her dreams about visiting Poland.

One day recently, not long after I left my former job to pursue my own practice, Mrs. Lo had a massive stroke. I talked to the Boss regularly. We discussed hospice, and the Boss agreed to that. "I just don't want her to leave my side," the Boss told me. "I don't want her to have to leave her apartment." I promised her that her mom would stay right there.

I visited Mrs. Lo a few days later. Other relatives were there, and Mrs. Lo was lying in her bed, smiling, mumbling a bit, and staring ahead. The Boss seemed very calm. After my requisite stethoscope to the chest, and after discussing with her what may come next in the dying process, the Boss looked at me and said, "Doctor, thank you so much for coming. Now I know that she'll be OK."

Mrs. Lo died a few days later, in her midnineties, in her own bed, her daughter by her side, free of pain or stress, likely thinking about the next car ride and her pending trip to Poland. Medicare paid very little for her care in her final years; she was a bargain for the system. The Boss innately understood the dangers of excess. She went cheap. So many others of my patients and families squander more Medicare dollars in a week than the Boss incurred in a decade. But the Boss considered herself just as thorough and loving as those other patients and families. She wanted the best for her mom. And she delivered on her word.

As a doctor who tries very hard to push my patients off the train of thorough, I know how difficult that is in our current environment. My patients read the papers, watch TV, surf the Internet, talk to friends and medical "experts," are privy to the many "breakthroughs" and "advances" that may help them if they just keep at it. Many buy into the specialized model of care that is so widely revered in this country. The hospital is clearly where most think they need to be if they are very sick, even if aspects of hospitalization frighten them. Many are suspicious of medicines, but want their numbers to look good, are afraid to stop their pills and supplements, believe in ample screening and testing especially if suggested by specialists or other smart people they know (even TV doctors), and cannot shake the idea that cure is possible for nuisance problems and for the inevitable symptoms of aging. Many would rather chase miracles than accommodate, exercise, and work hard at self-improvement.

Even if you incent a doctor like me to do less, which is what so many reforms are attempting, there is no chance of success unless Medicare changes its rules and payments that currently push my patients down a road of aggressive care that even the best of us cannot curtail. In the end, when financial incentives guide our elderly toward a path that emphasizes palliative medical care to enhance dignity and function, rather than down the costly precipice of high-cost medical aggression that swallows so many of my patients now, I know that people will be happier and healthier. Clinical studies, and the whole of my experience, demonstrate that the elderly do not want to be tossed into the caldron of medical excess when intervention is hopeless. Most of my patients seek comfort in their later years. And comfort comes cheap. It is hard to extirpate our medical falsehoods when they are so pervasive in society. But if Medicare changed course and nudged people in a different direction, then our medical landscape would be so much more beautiful and affordable.

If we intelligently curb care by allowing patients to make reasonable choices, we are not only going to save Medicare, but we will also be saving their lives. A thorough medical system need not bankrupt the insurance that finances it. In fact, the most thorough system that we can build for our elderly would be inexpensive, humane, and lifesaving. With just a sprinkle of political will, and a whiff of common sense, the answer sits upon our stoops. It is time to open up the door and take a look.

# ENDNOTES

1    http://www.thedailybeast.com/articles/2014/04/29/the-health-care-system-is-so-broken-it-s-time-for-doctors-to-strike.html

2    http://www.thedailybeast.com/articles/2014/04/14/how-being-a-doctor-became-the-most-miserable-profession.html

3.  Goodwin, "Geriatrics and the Limits of Modern Medicine," *New England Journal of Medicine* 340, no. 16 (1999): 1283-85.

4.  Shannon Brownlee, *Overtreated* (City: Bloomsbury Press, 2007), 199.

5.  Schwartz, "Enthusiasm for Cancer Screening in the United States," *Journal of the American Medical Association* (2004): 71-78.

6.  Paul Starr, *The Social Transformation of American Medicine* (New York: Basic Books, Inc., 1982), 280-86.

7.  *New York Times,* February 7, 1965, 57.

8.  Ward, *JAMA* (February 1965): 125.

9.  *New York Times,* May 12, 1965, 21.

10. Keim, *The New Republic* (February 13, 1965): 11.

11. Starr, *Social Transformation,* 369-78.

12. *JAMA* (February 1965): 17.

13. *New York Times,* August 5, 1965, 1.

14. *US News and World Report* (July 5, 1965): 26-28.

15. Starr, *Social Transformation,* 376-78.

16. Srestha, "The Changing Demographic Profile of the United States," *Congressional Research Services,* 2011, www.fas.for/sgp/crs/misc/rl32701.pdf.

17. *Alzheimer's Association,* www.alz.org.

18. www.medicalnewstoday.com/release/143784.pdf.

19. Ira Byock, *The Best Care Possible* (New York, Avery, 2012), 253.

20. www.cbo.gov/sites/default/files/cbofiles/attachments/12-01-medicarepartd.pdf.

21.  John Abramson, *Overdosed America* (New York, Harpers, 2008), 244-49.

22.  Rugg, "2011 Long Term Budget Outlook," *Congressional Budget Office*, 2011,.

23.  www.statistica.com/248073/distribution-of-medicare-spending-by-service-type/.

24.  www.medpac.gov/documents/June12/databookentirereport.pdf, 1-24.

25.  Boodman, "The 1% Solution," *Washington Post*, October 8, 2013, E1.

26.  RS Morrison, "When Too Much is Too Little," *New England Journal of Medicine* 335, no. 23 (1996): 1755-59.

27.  ES Fisher, "Medical Care—Is More Always Better?" *New England Journal of Medicine* 349, no. 17 (2003): 1665-67.

28.  Mitka, "Too Few Old Patients in Cancer Trials: Experts Say Disparity Affects Research Results and Care," *JAMA* 290 (2003): 27-28.

29.  Nortin Hadler, *Rethinking Aging* (Chapel Hill,: University of North Carolina Press, 2011), 190.

30.  Brownlee, *Overtreated*, 237.

31.  John Abramson, *Overdosed America*, (City: Harpers Collins Publishers, 2011), 183.

32.  Teno, "Medical Care Inconsistent with Patients' Treatment Goals," *Journal of the American Geriatric Society* 50 (2002): 496-500.

33.  PA Singer, "Quality End-of-Life Care: Patients' Perspectives," *JAMA* 281 (1999) 163-68.

34.  AE Bernato, "Are Regional Variations in End-of-life Care Intensity Explained by Patient Preferences?" *Med Care* 45 (2007): 386-93.

35.  Pronovost, "Economics of End-of-life Care in the Intensive Care Unit," *Critical Care Medicine* 29, no. 2 (2001): 46-51.

36.  Unroe, "Resource Use in the Last Six Months of Life Among Medicare Beneficiaries with Heart Failure: 2000-7," *Archives of Internal Medicine* 171, no. 3 (2011): 196-203.

37.  Robert Duggan, *Breaking the Iron Triangle* (City: Wisdom Well Press, 2012), 80.

38.  Hoover, "Medical Expenditures During the Last Year of Life," <u>Health Services Research</u>, 2002, 37(6): 1625-42

39.  Zhang, Baohui, "Health Care costs in the Last Week of Life: Association with End-of-life Conversations," <u>Archives of Internal Medicine</u>, 2009, 169(5): 480-85

40.  Lubitz, JD, "Trends in Medicare Payments in the Last Year of Life," <u>New England Journal of Medicine</u>, 1993, 328(15): 1092-96.

41.  Byock, <u>The Best Care Possible</u>, pg. 3

42.  Abramson, <u>Overdosed America</u>, pg. 247

43.  SHEP, "Prevention of Stroke by Antihypertensive Drug Treatment in Older Persons with Isolated Systolic Hypertension," <u>JAMA</u>, 1991, 165: 3255-64

44.  Hadler, <u>Rethinking Aging</u>, pg 13.

45.  Hadler, Nortin, <u>The Last Well Person</u>,2009, McGill-Queen's University Press, pg. 146

46.  Abramson, <u>Overdosed America</u>, pg, 103.

47.  Als-Neilson, "Association of Funding and Conclusions in Randomized Drug Trials," <u>JAMA</u>, 2003, 290: 921-28

48.  Chowdry, "Relationships Between Authors of Clinical Practice Guidelines and the Pharmaceutical Industry," <u>JAMA</u>, 2002, 287: 612-17.

49.  Brownlee, <u>Overtreated</u>, pg. 222-8.

50.  Boderheim, "Uneasy Alliance: Clinical Investigators and the Pharmaceutical Industry," <u>New England Journal of Medicine</u>, 2002, 32: 1539-44.

51.  Abramson, <u>Overdosed America</u>, pg. 115.

52.  Hohnloser, SH, "Incidence of Stroke in Paroxysmal vs. Sustained Afib in Patients Taking Oral Anticoagulation or Combined Antiplatelet Therapy," <u>Journal of the American College of Cardiology</u>, 2007, 50: 2156-61

53.  Mant, J, "Coumadin vs. Aspirin for Afib in the Elderly," <u>Lancet</u>, 2007, 370: 497-51

54. Ebell, M, "Chosing between Warfarin and Aspirin Therapy for Patients with Atrial Fibrillation," American Family Physician, June 2005, 71(12): 2348-50.

55. Fihn, SD, "The Risk for and Severity of Bleeding Complications in Elderly Patients Treated with Warfarin," Annals of Internal Medicine, 1996, 124 (11): 970-9

56. Gomes, T, "Rates of Hemorrhage During Warfarin Therapy for Atrial Fibrillation," CMAJ, 2013, 185: E121-27

57. The Stroke Prevention in Atrial Fibrillation Investigators, "Bleeding duing Anti-thrombotic Therapy in Patients with Atrial Fibrillation," Arch Intern Med, February 26, 1996, 156(4): 409-16.

58. Gage, BF, "Risk of Osteoporotic Fracture in Elderly Patients Taking Warfarin," Archives of Internal Medicine, 2006, 166: pg. 241

59. Powers, "Measuring Blood Pressure for Decision Making and Quarterly Reporting: Where and How Many Measures," Annals of Internal Medicine, 2011, 154: 781-85

60. Washington Post, June 4, 2013, pg. E1.

61. Ovbiagele, "Level of Systolic Blood Pressure within the Normal Range and Risk of Recurrent Stroke," JAMA, 2011, 306: 2137-44

62. Cooper, "Tight Blood Pressure Control and Cardiovascular Outcomes Among Hypertensive Patients with Diabetes and CAD," JAMA, 2010, 304: 61-8

63. Law, MR "Use of Blood Pressure Lowering Drugs in the Prevention of Cardiovascular Disease," British Medical Journal, 2009, 338: 1665

64. Messerli, FN, "Dogma Disputed: Can Aggressively Lowering Blood Pressure in Hypertensive Patients with CAD be Dangerous," Annals of Internal Medicine, 2006, 144; 884-93

65. Kovesdy, C, "Blood Pressure and Mortality in US Veterans with Chronic Kidney Disease," Annals of Internal Medicine, 2013, 159(4): 233-42

66. Hadler, Rethinking Aging, pg 45,48

67. Boutitie, F "J-shaped Relationship Between Blood Pressure and Mortality in Hypertensive Patients," <u>Annals of Internal Medicine</u>, 2002, 136(6): 438-48

68. Bangalor, MD, "What is the Optimal Blood Pressure in Patients after Acute Coronary Syndromes?," <u>Circulation</u>, 2010, 122: 142-5

69. Myers, M, "Overtreatment of Hypertension in the Community?" <u>American Journal of Hypertension</u>, 1996, 9(5): 419-25

70. Lernfelt, B, "Overtreatment of Hypertension in the Elderly?" <u>Journal of Hypertension</u>, 1990, 8(5): 483-90

71. Butt, "The Risk of Hip Fracture After Initiating Antihypertensive Drugs in the Elderly," <u>Archives of Internal Medicine</u>, 2012, 172: 1739-44

72. ADVANCE Collaborative Group, "Intense Blood Glucose Control and Vascular Outcomes in Patients with Type 2 Diabetes," <u>New England Journal of Medicine</u>, 2008, 358: 2560-71

73. Kelly, "Systemic Review: Glucose Control and Cardiovascular Disease in type 2 Diabetes," <u>Annals of Internal Medicine</u>, 2009, 151: 394-407

74. Duckworth, "Glucose Control and Vascular Complications in Veterans with Type 2 Diabetes," <u>New England Journal of Medicine</u>, 2009, 360: 129-39

75. Mitka, "Aggressive Glycemic Control Might Not be the Best Choice for all Diabetic Patients," <u>JAMA</u>, 303 (10): 1137-46

76. The Action to Control Cardiovascular Risk in Diabetes Study Group, "Effects of Intense glucose Lowering in Type 2 Diabetes," <u>New England Journal of Medicine</u>, 2008, 358: 2545-50

77. Whitner, "Hypoglycemic Episodes and Risk of Dementia in Patients with Type 2 Diabetes," <u>JAMA</u>, 2009, 301: 1565-71

78. Meinert, CL, "A Study of the Effects of Hypoglycemic Agents on Vascular Complications in Patients with Adult Onset Diabetes," <u>Diabetes</u>, 1970, 19: 789-830

79. Yau, CK, "Glycolylated Hemoglobin and Functional Decline in Community Dwelling Nursing Home Eligible Elderly Adults with Diabetes," <u>Journal of the American Geriatrics Society</u>, 2012, 60: 1215-21

80.  Aronow, W, "Oral Sulfonylurea and Cardiovascular Mortality," Geriatrics, 2004, 59(9): 45

81.  Simpson, S, "Dose-response Relationship Between Sulfonylurea Drugs and Mortality in Type 2 Diabetes: A Population Based Cohort Study," CMAJ, 2006, 174(2): 169-74.

82.  Hadler, Rethinking Aging, pp 34-37

83.  Lipscombe, "Thiazolidinediones and Cardiovascular Outcomes in Older Patients with Diabetes," JAMA, 2007, 298(22): 2634-43

84.  Kastelen, J, "Simvastatin with or without Ezetimine in Familial Hypercholesterolemia," New England Journal of Medicine, 2008, 358: 1431-43

85.  Dach, J, "Cholesterol Lowering Drugs for the Elderly, a Very Bad Idea," www.drdach.com/cholesterol_statin_elderly.html, 2008

86.  Rifkin, Erik, The Illusion of Certainty, Springer Press, 2007, pg. 89

87.  Abramson, Overdosed America, pp 14-16, p 145

88.  Hadler, The Last Well Person, pg 36

89.  Hadler, Rethinking Aging, pg 28

90.  Reiner, Z, "Statins in the Primary Prevention of Cardiovascular Disease," National Review of Cardiology, 2013, 10(8): 453-64

91.  http://www.medscape.com/viewarticle/814152

92.  Hadler, Rethinking Aging, pg 121

93.  Hadler, The Last Well Person, pg. 162

94.  Abramson, Overdosed America, pg 213

95.  Welch, Over-Diagnosed, pg 27

96.  Wells, GA, "Alendronate for the primary and secondary prevention of osteoporotic fractures in Postmenopausal Women," Cochrane Database of Systematic Review, 2008.

97.  Schneider, JP, "Bisphsphonates and low-impact femoral fractures: Current Evidence on alendronate fracture risk," Geriatrics, January 2009, 64(1): 18-23.

98.  Brownlee, Overtreated, pg 181

99.  Abramson, Overdosed America, pg. 104

100. Birks J. Cholinesterase inhibitors for Alzheimer's disease. <u>Cochrane Database Syst Rev</u>. 2006.

101. Kavirajan, H, "Efficacy and adverse effects of cholinesterase inhibitors and memantine in vascular dementia: a meta-analysis of randomised controlled trials," <u>The Lancet Neurology</u>, September, 2007, 6(9): 782-92.

102. Winblad B, "A 1-year, randomized, placebo-controlled study of donepezil in patients with mild to moderate AD," <u>*Neurology*</u> 2001;57:489-95

103. Howard, "Donepezil and Memantine for Moderate Severe Alzheimer's Disease," <u>New England Journal of Medicine</u>, 2012, 366: 893-903

104. Lanctot, K, "Efficacy and safety of cholinesterase inhibitors in Alzheimer's disease: a meta-analysis," <u>CMAJ</u> *September 16, 2003 vol. 169 no. 6*

105. Raina, P, "Effectiveness of Cholinesterase Inhibitors and Memantine for Treating Dementia: Evidence Review for a Clinical Practice Guideline,"<u>Annals of Internal Medicine</u>, 4 March 2008, 148(5): 379-97.

106. Schneider, L, "Lack of Evidence for the Efficacy of Memantine in Mild Alzheimer Disease," <u>Arch Neurol</u>. 2011;68(8):991-998.

107. Areosa SA, "Memantine for dementia," <u>Cochrane Database Syst Rev</u>. 2005;(3)

108. Searing, L, "A Daily Dose of Vitamin E May Slow Early Alzheimer's Disease," <u>The Washington Post</u>, January 4, 2014, pg. E3. This study compared Vitamin E to Namenda, and found that Namanda had no impact on function while Vitamin E did.

109. Howard, "Donepezil and Memantine for Moderate Severe Alzheimer's Disease," <u>New England Journal of Medicine</u>, 2012, 366: 893-903

110. Middleton, "Activity Energy Expenditure and Incident of Cognitive Impairment in Older Adults," <u>Archives of Internal Medicine</u>, 2011, 171: 1251-57

111.   Russian, EB, "Exercise is Associated with Reduced Risk for Incident Dementia Among Persons 64 Years Old and Older," <u>Annals of Internal Medicine</u>, 2006, 144: 73-81

112.   Laurin, D, "Physicial Activity and Risk of Cognitive Impairment and Dementia in Elderly Person," <u>Archives of Neurology</u>, 2001, 58: 498-504

113.   Hadler, <u>Rethinking Aging</u>, pg 168

114.   http://www.ahrp.org/cms/content/view/813/56. Also, most other studies cited show the high side effect profile and dropout rate.

115.   Gill, S, "Syncope and its Consequences in Patients with Dementia receiving Cholinesterase Inhibitors," <u>Archives of Internal Medicine</u>, 2009, 169: 86 7-73

116.   Brownlee, <u>Overtreated</u>, pg 186

117.   Donohue, J, "A Decade of Direct-to-consumer Advertising on Prescription Drugs," <u>New England Journal of Medicine</u>, 2007, 357: 673-81

118.   Orlowski, "The Effects of Pharmaceutical Firms on Physician Prescribing Patterns," <u>Chest</u>, 1992, 102: 270-77

119.   Dana, "A Social Science Perspective on Gifts to Physicians from Industry," <u>JAMA</u>, 2003, 290: 252

120.   Wazana, A, "Physicians and the Pharmaceutical Industry," <u>JAMA</u>, 2000, 283(3): 373-8

121.   Abramson, <u>Overdosed America</u>, pg. 105

122.   Adair, F, "Do Drug Samples Influence Resident Prescribing Behavior?" <u>American Journal of Medicine</u>, 2005, 118: 881-4

123.   Abramson, <u>Overdosed America</u>, pg 101

124.   Brownlee, <u>Overtreated</u>, pg 219 ****check this to make sure not Welch

125.   Yu-xio Yang, "Long Term Proton Pump Inhibitor Therapy and Risk of Hip Fracture," <u>JAMA</u>, 2006, 296: 2947-53

126.   Diem, SJ, "Use of Antidepressants and Rate of Hip Bone Loss in Older Women," <u>Archives of Internal Medicine</u>, 2007, 167: 1240-45

127. Hadler, <u>Rethinking Aging</u>, pg 165

128. HOPE-TOO Trial Investigators, "Long Term Vitamin E Supplements in Patients with Vascular Disease or Diabetes," <u>JAMA</u>, 2005, 293: 138-47

129. Albert, CM, "Effect of Folic Acid and B Vitamins on Risk of Cardiovascular Events and Total Mortality Among Females at High Risk for Cardiovascular Disease," <u>JAMA</u>, 2008, 299: 2027-31

130. Myura, "Efficacy of Vitamin and Anti-oxidant Supplements in Prevention of Cardiovascular Disease," <u>BMJ</u>, 2013, 346: F10

131. Klein, "Vitamin E and the Risk of Prostate Cancer: The Selenium and Vitamin E Cancer Prevention Trial," <u>JAMA</u>, 2011, 306: 1549-55

132. Searing, L, "A Daily Dose of Vitamin E May Slow Early Alzheimer's Disease," <u>The Washington Post</u>, January 4, 2014, pg. E3.

133. Ernst, E, "The Risk-Benefit Profile of Commonly Used Herbal Therapies," <u>Annals of Internal Medicine</u>, 2002, 136(1): 42-53

134. Bolland, MJ, "Vascular Events in Healthy Older Women Receiving Calcium Supplementation," 2008, http://www.bmj.com/content/336/7638/262

135. Hadler, <u>Last Well Person</u>, pg 154

136. Reid, I, "Calcium Supplements with or without Vitamin D and Risk of Cardiovascular Events," <u>BMJ</u>, 2011, http://www.bmj.com/content/342/bmj.d2040

137. Seeman, E, "Evidence that Calcium Supplements Reduce Fracture risk is Lacking," <u>CJASN</u>, Jaunary 2010, 5: S53-11.

138. Bolland, MJ, ""Calcium Supplements and Fracture Prevention," <u>New England Journal of Medicine</u>, January 2014, 370: 386-88

139. Bolland, MJ, "Calcium Supplements with or without Vitamin D and Risk of Cardiovascular Events: Reanalysis of the Women's Health Initiative," <u>BMJ</u>, 2011, 342: d2040.

140. Kwak, S, "Efficacy of Omega-3 Fatty Acid Supplements in the Secondary Prevention of Cardiovascular Disease," <u>Archives of Internal Medicine</u>, 2012, 175(9): 686-94

141. Risk and Prevention Study Collaborative Group, "N-3 Fatty Acids in Patients with Multiple Cardiovascular Risk Factors," New England Journal of Medicine, 2013, 368: 1800-08

142. Brasky, TM, "Plasma Phospholipid Fatty Acids and Prostate Cancer Risk in the SELECT Trial," Journal of the National Cancer Institute, 2013, 105(15): 1132-41

143. Multiple trials of Omega-3 acids have been conducted with varying results, some of which have different doses and examine different populations. None show dramatic improvement, but some do show a cardiac benefit in certain circumstances.

144. Seshasai, "Effect of Aspirin on Vascular and Nonvascular Outcomes: Meta-analysis of Randomized Controlled Trials," Archives of Internal Medicine, 2012, 172: 206-16

145. Eliseo Guallar, MD, DrPH "Enough Is Enough: Stop Wasting Money on Vitamin and Mineral Supplements," Annals of Internal Medicine, December 17, 2013, 159(12): 850-1. See accompanying studies in the same issue that look in depth at multi-vitamin supplementation.

146. Mursu, J, "Dietary Supplements and Mortality Rate in Older Women: The Iowa Women's Health Study," Archives of Internal Medicine, 2011, 171: 1625-33

147. Quato, DM, "Use of Prescription and OTC Medicines and Dietary Supplements Among Older Adults in the United States," JAMA, 2008, 300: 2867-78

148. Bjelakovic, "Mortality in Randomized Trials of Antioxidant Supplements for Primary and Secondary Prevention," JAMA, 2007, 297: 842-57

149. Cha, A, "Study Questions Antioxidant Use in Cancer Patients," the Washington Post, January 30, 2014, pg. A2.

150. Bjelakovic G, "Antioxidant supplements to prevent mortality,". JAMA. Sept 18, 2013; 310:1178-9.

151. Heart Protection Study Collaboration Group. "MRC/BHF Heart Protection Study of antioxidant vitamin supplementation in

20 536 high-risk individuals: a randomised placebo-controlled trial," Lancet. 2002;360:23-33

152. Kaptchuck, TJ, "Placebo Without Deception," Plosone, 2010, http://www.plosone.org/article/info%3Adoi%2F10.1371%2Fjournal. pone.0015591

153. Barrett, "Placebo Effects and the Common Cold: A Randomized Controlled Trial," Annals of Family Medicine, 2011, 9: 312-27

154. Abramson, Overdiagnosed America, pg 127, 140

155. Guallar, E, "Controversy Over Clinical Guidelines: Listen to the Evidence, not the Noise," Annals of Internal Medicine, March 4, 2014, 160(5): 361-2.

156. See for example, www.kaiserpermanente.org/html/cpp_cod/ clinicalguidelines.html

157. Available in the Northern Maryland Collaborative Care handbook.

158. Gurwitz, JH, "Incidence and Preventability of Adverse Drug Events among Older Persons," JAMA, 2003, 289(9): 1107-16

159. Voelker, R "Common Drugs Can Harm Elderly Patients," JAMA, 2009, 302(6): 614

160. Routledge, P, "Adverse Drug Reactions in Elderly Patients," British Journal of Clinical Pharmacology, 2004, 57(2): 121-26

161. Kurfees, JF, "Drug Interactions in the Elderly," Journal of Family Practice, 1987, 25(5): 471-85

162. Brownlee, Overtreatment, pg. 274

163. Starfield, B, "Is US Health Really the Best in the World," JAMA, 2000, 284(4): 483-85

164. Deyo, RA, "Cascade Effects of Medical Technology," Annual Review of Public Health, 2002, 23: 23-44

165. Brownlee, Overtreated, pg 158

166. Brownlee, Overtreated, pg 144

167. Welch, Overdiagnosed, pg 35

168. Brownlee, Overtreated, pg 105

169.  See especially Welch, <u>Overdiagnosed</u> and Rifkin, <u>The Illusion of Certainty</u>

170.  Davies, B, "Rethinking the Value of the Annual Exam," <u>ACP Internist</u>, January, 2010

171.  Hadler, <u>Rethinking Aging</u>, pg 67

172.  Welch, <u>Overdiagnosed</u>, pg 49

173.  Andriole, "Mortality Results from a Randomized Prostate Cancer Screening Trial," <u>New England Journal of Medicine</u>, 2009, 360: 1310-19

174.  Welch, HG "Prostate Cancer Diagnosis and Treatment After the Introduction of PSA Screening, 1986-2005," <u>Journal of National Cancer Institute</u>, 2009, 101 (19): 1325-29

175.  Brownlee, <u>Overtreated</u>, pg 200

176.  Link, "Benefits and Harms of PSA Screening for Prostate Cancer: An Evidence Update for the US Preventive Task Force," <u>Annals of Internal Medicine</u>, 2008, 149: 192-99

177.  Ibid

178.  Heijnsdijk, "Quality of Life Effect of PSA Screening," <u>New England Journal of Medicine</u>, 2012, 367: 595-605

179.  Fang, F, "Immediate Risk for Cardiovascular Events and Suicide Following a Prostate Cancer Diagnosis," <u>Journal of National Cancer Institute</u>, 2010, 102(5): 307-14

180.  Smith, DP, "Quality of Life Three Years After Diagnosis of Localized Prostate Cancer," <u>BMJ</u>, 2009, 339, http://www.ncbi.nlm.nih.gov/pubmed/19945997

181.  Hadler, <u>The Last Well Person</u>, pg. 99

182.  Welch, <u>Overdiagnosed</u>, Hadler <u>Last Well Person</u>, and Abramson <u>Overdiagnosed</u> all talk about futility of cancer treatment in extending life.

183.  www.uspreventiveservicestaskforce.gov

184.  Bleyer, "Effect of Three Decades of Screening Mammograms on Breast Cancer Incidence," <u>New England Journal of Medicine</u>, 2012, 367: 1998-2005

185.   Welch, HG, "Over Diagnosis of Mammogram Screening: The Question if not Whether but How Often it Occurs," <u>BMJ</u>, 2009, 339: 182-3

186.   Welch, HG, "Screening Mammography: A Long Run for a Short Ride," <u>New England Journal of Medicine</u>, 2010, 363: 1276-80

187.   Phillips, KA, "Putting the Risk of Breast Cancer into Perspective," <u>New England Journal of Medicine</u>, 1999, 340(2): 141-4

188.   Zahl, DH, "The Natural History of Invasive Breast Cancer Detected by Screening Mammography," <u>Archives of Internal Medicine</u>, 2008, 168(21): 2311-15

189.   Kolata, G, "Vest Study Casts Doubt on Value of Mammogram," <u>The New York Times</u>, February 12, 2014. http://www.nytimes.com/2014/02/12/health/study-adds-new-doubts-about-value-of-mammograms.html?_r=0

190.   Welch, H, "Breast Cancer Screenings: What we Still Don't Know," <u>The New York Times</u>, December 30, 2013.

191.   Monsees, B, 'Weighing the Value of Mammogram," <u>The New York Times</u>, January 2, 2014.

192.   Walter, L, "Cancer Screening in Elderly Patients," <u>Journal of the American Medical Association</u>, June 2001, 285(21): pp. 2750-56.

193.   Smith-Bindman, R, "Is Screening Mammography Effective in Elderly Women?," <u>American Journal of Medicine</u>, February 2000, 108(2): pp. 112-9.

194.   Lerman, C" Psychological and Behavior Implications of Abnormal Mammograms," <u>Annals of Internal Medicine</u>, 1991, 114(8): 657-61

195.   Brewer, NT, "The Long Term Effects of False Positive Mammograms," <u>Annals of Internal Medicine</u>, 2007, 146(7): 502-10

196.   http://well.blogs.nytimes.com/2012/05/09/new-cautions-about-long-term-use-of-bone-drugs/?_r=0

197.http://www.health.harvard.edu/newsletters/Harvard_Womens_Health_Watch/2008/November/Whats_the_story_with_Fosamax. See also references from chapter 2 about Fosamax.

198. Brownlee, <u>Overtreated</u>, pg 213

199. Gourlay, "Bone Density Testing Intervals and Transition to Osteoporosis in Older Women," <u>New England Journal of Medicine</u>, 2012, 366: 225-32

200. Herndon, "Implications of Expanded Disease Definitions: The Case of Osteoporosis," <u>Health Affairs</u>, 2007, 26: 1702-11

201. Hadler, <u>The Last Well Person</u>, pg 72

202. Span, P, "Too many Colonoscopies in the Elderly," <u>The New York Times</u>, March 12, 2013.

203. Wilson, J, "Colon Cancer Screening in the Elderly: When do we Stop?" Trans AmClinClimatol Assoc, 2010, 121: 94-103.

204. Pastorino, V, "Early Lung Cancer Detection with Spiral CT and Positron Emission Tomography in Heavy Smokers: 2 Year Results," <u>Lancet</u>, 2003, 362: 593-7

205. NLST Research Team, "Reduced Lung-Cancer Mortality with Low-dose CT Screening," <u>New England Journal of Medicine</u>, August 10, 2011, 365:395-409.

206. De Koning, H, "Benefits and Harms of Computed Tomography Lung Cancer Screening Strategies: A Comparative Modeling Study for the US Preventive Services Task Force," <u>Annals of Internal Medicine</u>, March 4, 2014, 160(5): 311-20.

207. Patz, EF, "Overdiagnosis in low-dose computed tomography screening for lung cancer," <u>JAMA Internal Medicine</u>, February 1, 2014, 174(2): 269-74.

208. Fein, "Clinical Practice: The Solitary Pulmonary Nodule," <u>New England Journal of Medicine</u>, 2003, 348: 2535-47

209. MacMahon, H, "Guidelines for Management of Small Pulmonary Nodules Detected on CT Scans," <u>Radiology</u>, 2005, 237: 395-406

210. Welch, <u>Overdiagnosed</u>, pg 67

211. Welch, HG, "Overdiagnosis in Cancer," <u>J. Natl Cancer Inst</u>, May 5, 2010, 102(9): 605-13.

212. Berrington de Gonzalez, A, "Low Dose Lung CT screening before age 55: Estimates of the Mortality Reduction Required to Outweigh the Radiation-induced Cancer Risk," J. Med Screening, 2008, 15(3): 153-8.

213. Hanh, P, Baltimore Sun, March 29, 2013, pg. 17

214. Welch, Overdiagnosed, pg 144

215. Hadler, Rethinking Aging, pg. 50

216. Welch, Overdiagnosed, pg. 114

217. Brownlee, Overtreated, pg 150, 158, 166

218. Welch, Overdiagnosed, pg. 36

219. Bruyere, O, "Radiologic Features Poorly Predict Clinical Outcome in Knee Osteoarthritis," Scandinavian Journal of Rheumatology, 2002, 31(1): 13-16

220. England, "Incidental Meniscal Findings on Knee MRI in Middle Age and Elderly Persons," New England Journal of Medicine, 2008, 359: 1108-15

221. Redberg, R, "We are Giving Ourselves Cancer," The New York Times, January 31, 2014, pg. A27.

222. Welch, Overdiagnosed, pg. 47

223. Brownlee, Overtreated, pg. 149

224. Jarvik, J, "Diagnostic Evaluation of Lower Back Pain with Emphasis on Imaging," Annals of Internal Medicine, 2002, 37(7): 586-97

225. Roudsari, B, "Lumbar Spine MRI for Low Back Pain: Indications and Yield," AJR Am J Roetgenol, 2010, 195(3): 550-9

226. El Barzouhi, A, "Magnetic Resonance Imaging in Follow-up Assessment of Sciatica," New England Journal of Medicine, 2013, 368: 999-1007

227. Chou, R, "Diagnostic Imaging for Low Back Pain: Advice for High-Value Health Care From the American College of Physicians," Annals of Internal Medicine, February 1, 2011, 154(3): 181-9.

228. Pengel LH, "Acute low back pain: systematic review of its prognosis,: BMJ. 2003; 327:323.

229. Chou R, "Imaging strategies for low-back pain: systematic review and meta-analysis," Lancet. 2009; 373:463.-72.

230. Webster BS, "Relationship of early magnetic resonance imaging for work-related acute low back pain with disability and medical utilization outcomes," J Occup Environ Med. 2010; 52:900.-7

231. Jensen, "MRI of the Lumbar Spine in People without Back Pain," New England Journal of Medicine, 1994, 331: 69-78

232. Videman, T, "Associations between Back Pain History and Lumbar MRI Findings," Spine, 2003, 28(6): 582-8

233. Choi, HJ, "Epidural Steroid Injection Therapy for Lower Back Pain," Int J TEchnol Assess Health Care, 2013, 29(3): 244-53

234. Chou, R, "Surgery for Lower Back Pain: A Review of the Evidence for an American Pain Society Clinical Practice Guideline," Spine, 2009, 34(10): 1094-1109

235. Radcliff, K, "Epidural steroid injections are associated with less improvement in patients with lumbar spinal stenosis: a subgroup analysis of the Spine Patient Outcomes Research Trial," Spine, February 15, 2013, 38(4): 279-91

236. Brody, J, "The Treadmill's Place in Evaluating Hearts," The New York Times, July 29, 2008.

237. Arbab-Saden, A, "Stress Tesing and Non-invasive Coronary Angiogrophy in Patients with Suspected Coronary Artery Disease," Heart International, February, 2012, 7(1): e2.

238. Capewell, "Will Screening Individuals High Risk of Cardiovascular Events Deliver Large Benefits?" BMJ, 2005, 337: 783, which is a medical repudiation of an article stating the opposite

239. Fein, David. http://www.theplc.net/Cardiac_Stress_Tests.html

240. Skinner, J, "Is Technological Change in Medicine Always Worth It: The Case of Myocardial Infarction?" Health Affairs, 2006, 25(2): w34-47

241. Tu, J, "Use of Cardiac Procedures and Outcomes in Elderly Patients with Myocardial Infarction in the United States and Canada," New England Journal of Medicine, 1997, 336(21): 1500-5

242. Abramson, <u>Overdosed America</u>, pg. 172

243. Brownlee, <u>Overtreated</u>, Pg 99

244. Boden, WE, "Optimal Medical Therapy with or without PCI for Stable CAD," <u>New England Journal of Medicine</u>, 2007, 356: 1503-16, shows that adding revascularization to medicines and lifestyle changes does not improve outcomes.

245. Pfisterer, M "Outcomes of Elderly Patients with Chronic Symptomatic Coronary Artery Disease with an Invasive vs. Optimized Medical Treatment Strategy," <u>JAMA</u>, 2003, 289(9): 1117-23

246. Henderson, "Seven Year Outcome in the RITA-2 Trial: Coronary Angioplasty vs. Medical Therapy," <u>Journal of the American College of Cardiology</u>, 2003, 42: 1161-70

247. Hadler, <u>The Last Well Person</u>, pp 27-9

248. Brownlee, <u>Overtreated</u>, pp. 101-2

249. Hadler, <u>Rethinking Aging</u>, pp. 54-5

250. Abramson, <u>Overdosed America</u>, pg. 172

251. Newman, "Longitudinal Assessment of Neurocognitive Function after CABG," <u>New England Journal of Medicine</u>, 2003, 344(6): 395-402

252. Thorsteinsdottir, B, "Dialysis in the Frail Elderly—A Current Ethical Problem, an Impending Ethical Crisis," <u>Journal of General Internal Medicine</u>, 2013

253. Tamura, "Functional Status of Elderly Adults Before and After Initiation of Dialysis," <u>New England Journal of Medicine</u>, 2009, 361: 1539-47, showing a substantial decline in status on nursing home residents on dialysis

254. Arnold, "Dialysis in Frail Elders—a Role for Palliative Care," <u>New England Journal of Medicine</u>, 2009, 361: 1597-8

255. Black, NA, "The Effectiveness of Surgery for Stress Incontinence in Women," <u>British Journal of Urology</u>, 1996, 78(4): 497-510

256. <u>Tell Me More</u>, National Public Radio, August 14, 2013

257. Mark-Clarfield, A, "The Decreasing Prevalence of Reversible DementiasAn Updated Meta-analysis," <u>Arch Intern Med.</u>, October 13, 2003;163(18):2219-2229.

258. Starfield, B, "The Effects of Specialist Supply on a Population's Health." <u>Health Affairs</u>, 2005, 97-107

259. Macinko, "Quantifying the Health Benefit of Primary Care Physician Supply in the United States," <u>Int J. Health Serv</u>, 2007, 37(1): 111-26

260. Wennberg, JE, "Executive Summary of Tracking the Care of Patients with Severe Chronic Illness: The Dartmouth Atlas of Health Care 2008," Hanover, NH, Dartmouth Institute for Policy and Clinical Practice, Center for Health Policy Research

261. Brownlee, <u>Overtreated</u>, pg. 36. See also Wennberg, JE, "Geography and the Debate Over Medicare Reform," <u>Health Affairs</u>, 2002.

262. Brownlee, <u>Overtreated</u>, pp 63, 67.

263. <u>Washington Post</u>, April 30, 2013, E5.

264. Carey, T, "The Outcomes and Costs of Care for Acute Low Back Pain Among Patients Seen by Primary Care Practitioners, Chiropractors, and Orthopedic Surgeons," <u>New England Journal of Medicine</u>, 1995, 333: 913-17

265. Rosenthal, E, "The $2.7 Trillion Medical Bill," <u>The New York Times</u>, June 1, 2013.

266. Hadler, <u>Rethinking Aging</u>, pg. 187

267. Brownlee, <u>Overtreatment</u>, pg. 81

268. Abramson, <u>Overdosed America</u>, pg. 50

269. Jacobson, M, "Does Reimbursement Influence Chemotherapy Treatment for Cancer Patients?" <u>Health Affairs</u>, 2006, 25(2): 437-43

270. Erikson, J, "Oncologists Cutting Back in Face of New Medicare Payment Formula," <u>Oncology Times</u>, 2004, 26(4): 4-8

271. Abramson, <u>Overdosed America</u>, pg. 83

272. Brownlee, <u>Overtreatment</u>, pp. 153, 265

273. Compton, M, "Changes in US Medical Students' Specialty Interests Over the Course of Medical School," <u>Journal of General Internal Medicine</u>, 2008, 23(7): 1095-1100

274. Bodenhemer, "Primary Care—Will it Survive?" <u>New England Journal of Medicine</u>, 2006, 355(9): 861-3

275.   Brandon, G, "How Medical Schools Consistently Cover up Their Primary Care Failures," <u>Medical Economics</u>, May 28, 2013

276.   Brownlee, <u>Overtreated</u>, pg 259

277.   Block, "Academia's Chilly Climate for Primary Care," <u>JAMA</u>, 1996, 206: 677-82

278.   Newton, "Trends in Career Choice by US Medical Schools," <u>JAMA</u>, 2007, 209: 1179-82

279.   Brownlee, <u>Overtreated</u>, pg. 259

280.   www.medscape.features/slideshow/compensation/2012

281.   McGann, P, "Quality Improvement Initiatives and Tools," AMDA Conference, March 23, 2013

282.   Glenn, B, "Why Aren't Primary Care Physicians more Ticked Off about the RUC?" <u>Medical Economics</u>, April 30, 2013

283.   Whoriskey, P, "Medical Panel Uses Data that Distorts Doctors' Pay," <u>The Washington Post</u>, July 21, 2013, pg. 1

284.   Studert, DM, "Claims, Errors, and Compensatory Payments in Malpractice Litigation," <u>New England Journal of Medicine</u>, 2006, 354: 2024-33

285.   Kahn-Fogel, N, "Hanging in the Balance: Health Dogma and the Debate over Malpractice Reform," <u>Journal of the National Medical Association</u>, 2010, 102(3): 254-6

286.   Golann, D, "Dropped Medical Malpractice Claims: Their Surprising Frequency Apparent Causes and Potential Remedies," <u>Health Affairs</u>, 2011, 30(7): 1343-50

287.   Carrier, E, "High Physician Concern about Malpractice Risk Predicts More Aggressive Diagnostic Testing in Office-based Practice," <u>Health Affairs</u>, 2013, 32(8): 1383-91

288.   Weisman, CS, "Practice Changes in Response to the Malpractice Litigation Climate: Results of a Physician Survey," <u>Medical Care</u>, 1989, 27(1): 16-24

289.   Studdart, D, "Defensive Medicine among High-risk Specialist Physicians in a Volatile Malpractice Environment," <u>JAMA</u>, 2005, 295(21): 2609-17

290.    Katz, D, "Emergency Physicians Fear of Malpractice in Evaluating Patients with Possible Acute Cardiac Ischemia," <u>Annals of Emergency Medicine</u>, 2005, 46(6): 525-33

291.    Birbeck, GL, "Do Malpractice Concerns, Payment Mechanisms, and Attitudes Influence Test Ordering Decisions?" <u>Neurology</u>, 2004, 62(1): 119-21

292.    Krist, "How Physicians Approach Prostate Cancer Before and After Losing a Law Suit," <u>Annals of Family Medicine</u>, 2007, 5: 120-7

293.    Klingman, D, "Measuring Defensive Medicine using Clinical Scenario Surveys," <u>Journal of Health Politics, Policy, and Law</u>, 1996, 2185-217

294.    Seabury, S, "On Average, Physicians Spend Nearly 11% of their 40 Year Careers with an Open, Unresolved Malpractice Claim," <u>Health Affairs</u>, 2013, 32(1): 111-15

295.    Silver, C, "The Poor State of Health Care Quality in the US: Is Malpractice Liability Part of the Problem or Part of the Solution," <u>Bepress Legal Series</u>, 2004, pg. 222.

296.    Kesselheim, A, "Characteristics of Physicians who Frequently Act as Expert Witnesses in Neurologic Birth Injury Litigation," <u>Obstetrics and Gynecology</u>, 2006, 108(2): 273-9

297.    Weintraub, M, "Expert Witness Testimony: An Update," <u>Neurology Clinics</u>, 1999, 17(2): 363-69

298.    Paul, S, "States, Physician Organizations, Courts Take on Unethical Medical Experts," <u>AAP News</u>, 2013, 34(2).

299.    Kesselheim, A, "Role of Professional Organizations in Regulating Physician Expert Witness Testimony," <u>JAMA</u>, 2007, 298(24): 2907-9

300.    www.medpac.gov\documents\june12\datebookentirereport.pdf, pp 1-24

301.    www.ncpssm.org/medicare/medicarefastfacts

302.    http://assets.aarp.org/rgcenter/health/fs149_medicare.pdf

303.    Brownlee, <u>Overtreatment</u>, pp 47, 52

304.    Kohn, L, "To Err is Human: Building a Safer Health System," 2000, National Academy Press

305.  Ehlenbach, WJ, "Association between Acute Care and Critical Illness Hospitalization and Cognitive Function in Older Adults," JAMA, 2010, 303(8): 763-7

306.  Witlox, "Delirium in Elderly Patients and the Risk of Post Discharge Mortality, Institutionalized, and Dementia," JAMA, 2010, 304: 443-51

307.  Wonsch, "Three Year Outcome for Medicare Beneficiaries who Survive Intensive Care," JAMA, 2010, 303: 849-60

308.  Walter, L, "Development and Validation of a Prognostic Index for Mortality in Older Adults after Hospitalization," JAMA, 2001, 285(23): 2987-94

309.  Hadler, Rethinking Aging, pg 193

310.  Meier, "High Short-term Mortality in Hospitalized Patients with Advanced Dementia: Lack of Benefit of Tube Feeding," Archives of Internal Medicine, 2001, 164(4): 594-99

311.  Curtis, LH, "Early and Long-term Outcome of Heart Failure in Elderly Persons, 2001-05," Archives of Internal Medicine, 2008, 168(22): 2481-85

312.  Pedone, "Elderly Patients with Cognitive Impairment have a High Risk for Functional Decline During Hospitalization," J. Gerontol A Biol Med Sci, 2005, 60(12): 1576-80

313.  Morton, C, "Hazards of Hospitalization of the Elderly," Annals of Internal Medicine, 1993, 118(3): 219-23

314.  Covinsky, KE, "Loss of Independence in Activities of Daily Living in Older Adults Hospitalized with Medical Illness: Increased Vulnerability with Age," Journal of the American Geriatrics Society, 2003, 51: 451-8

315.  Gill, "Hospitalization, Restricted Activity, and the Development of Disability among Older Persons," JAMA, 2004, 292(17): 2115-20

316.  Quach, "Risk of Infection Following a Visit to the Emergency Department: a Cohort Study," CMAJ, 2012, 184: E232-39

317.  Bernstein, L, "1 in 25 Hospital Patients gets an Infection during Treatment, CDC Reports," The Washington Post, March 27, 2014, pg. A3.

318.  Duggan, Robert, <u>Breaking the Iron Triangle</u>, Wisdom Well Press, 2012, pg. 77

319.  Kruse, RL, "Does Hospitalization Impact Survival After Lower Respiratory Infection in Nursing Home Residents?" <u>Medical Care</u>, 2004, 42: 860-70

320.  Loeb, M, "Effect of a Clinical Pathway to Reduce Hospitalization in Nursing Home Residents with Pneumonia," <u>JAMA</u>, 2006, 295: 2503-10

321.  Givens, JL, "Survival and Comfort After Treatment of Pneumonia in Advanced Dementia," <u>Archives of Internal Medicine</u>, 2011, 171: 217

322.  Byock, I, <u>The Best Care Possible</u>, pp. 107-9

323.  Longstrot, WT, "Intravenous Tissue Plasminogen Activator and Stroke in the Elderly," <u>American Journal of Emergency Medicine</u>, 2010, 28(3): 359-63

324.  Sharma, G, "Trends in End-of-life ICU Care Among Older Adults with Advanced Lung Cancer," <u>Chest</u>, 2008, 133(1): 72-8.

325.  Kelley, A, "Determinants of Medical Expenditures in the Last Six Months of Life," <u>Annals of Internal Medicine</u>, 2011, 154: 235-42

326.  Kaufman, S, "Making Longevity in an Aging Society: Linking Ethical Sensibility and Medicare Spending," <u>Medical Anthropology</u>, 2009, 28(4): 317-25

327.  Jennings, B, "Health Care Costs in End-of-life and Palliative Care: The Quest for Ethical Reform," <u>Journal of Social Work</u>, 2011, 7: 300-17

328.  Duggan, <u>Breaking the Iron Triangle</u>, pg. 80

329.  Brownlee, <u>Overtreated</u>, pg. 115

330.  Pritchard, "Influence of Patient Preferences and Local Health System Characteristics on the Place of Death," <u>Journal of the American Geriatrics Society</u>, 1995, 46: 1242-50

331.  See notes 10-14 in chapter 1

332.  Brownlee, <u>Overtreated</u>, pp49, 59, 113

333.  www.texmed.org/community_acquired_pneumonia.aspx

334.  Frick, KD, "Substitutive Hospital at Home for Older Persons: Effect on Costs," <u>American Journal of Managed Care</u>, 2009, 15(1): 49-56.

335. Byock, <u>The Best Care Possible</u>, pg. 233

336. http://www.baltimoresun.com/health/maryland-health/bal-total-compensation-for-maryland-hospital-ceos-and-presidents-20130816,0,1549191.htmlpage

337. http://www.aha.org/content/00-10/2010econcontrib.pdf

338. www.ogg.osu.edu/traditional-hospital-care-vs-ace-units-for-geriatric-patients/ 2009

339. Fox, MT, "Effectiveness of Acute Geriatric Unit Care using acute Care for elders Components: a Systematic Review and Met analysis," <u>Journal of the American Geriatrics Society</u>, 2012, 60(12): 2237-45

340. Counsell, S, "Effects of a Multicomponent Intervention on Functional Outcomes and Process of Care in Hospitalized Older Patients: a Randomized controlled Trial of Acute Care for Elders (ACE) in a Community Hospital," <u>Journal of the American Geriatrics Society</u>, 2000, 48(12): 1572-81

341. Flood, K, "Effect of an Acute Care for Elders Unit on costs and Thirty Day Readmissions," <u>JAMA</u>, 2013, 173(11): 981-7

342. www.holycrosshealth.org/seniors-emergency-centers

343. Hwang, U, "The Geriatric Emergency Department," <u>Journal of the American Geriatrics Society</u>, 2007, 55(11): 1873-6

344. Byock, <u>The Best Care Possible</u>, pp. 112, 230

345. Hadler, <u>Rethinking Aging</u>, pg 171

346. Walshe, K, "Regulating US Nursing Homes: Are We Learning from Experience?" <u>Health Affairs</u>, 2001, 20(6): 128-44

347. Troyer, J, "The Impact of Litigation on Nursing Home Quality," <u>Journal of Health Politics, Policy, and Law</u>, 2004, 29(1): 11-42

348. Gillick, M, "Rethinking the Role of Tube Feeds in Patients with Advanced Dementia," <u>New England Journal of Medicine</u>, 2000, 342(3): 206-10

349. Kau, M, "Long-term Follow-up of Consequences of PEG Tubes in Nursing Home Patients," <u>Digestive Disease and Science</u>, 1994, 39(4): 738-43

350.  Mitchell, S, "The Risk Factors and Impact on Survival of Feeding Tube Placement in Nursing Home Residents with Severe Cognitive Impairment," Archives of Internal Medicine, 1997, 157(3): 327-32

351.  Rubenstein, L, "Falls in the Nursing Home," Annals of Internal Medicine, 1994, 121(6): 442-51

352.  Lipsitz, L, "Cause and Correlates of Recurrent Falls in Ambulatory Frail Elderly," Journal of Gerontolgy, 1991, 46(4): 114-22

353.  Rubenstein, L, "Falls and Fall Prevention in the Nursing Home," Clinics in Geriatric Medicine, 1996, 12(4): 881-902

354.  Abramson, Overdosed America, pg. 218

355.  Cohen-Mansfield, J, "Turnover Among Nursing Home Staff: A Review," Nurse Manager, 1997, 28(5): 59-64

356.  Castle, N, "Staff Turnover and Quality of Care in Nursing Homes," Medical Care, 2005, 43(6): 616-26

357.  Harrington, C, "Nursing Home Staffing and its Relationship to Deficiencies," The Journal of Gerontology, 2000, 55(5): 278-87

358.  Kruse, RL, "Does Hospitalization Impact Survival After Lower Respiratory Infection in Nursing Home Residents?" Medical Care, 2004, 42: 860-70

359.  Loeb, M, "Effect of a Clinical Pathway to Reduce Hospitalization in Nursing Home Residents with Pneumonia," JAMA, 2006, 295: 2503-10

360.  Givens, JL, "Survival and Comfort After Treatment of Pneumonia in Advanced Dementia," Archives of Internal Medicine, 2011, 171: 217

361.  Gozalo, P, "End-of-life Transitions among Nursing Home Residents with Cognitive Issues," New England Journal of Medicine, 2011, 365: 1212-21

362.  Forster, AJ, "The Incidence and Severity of Adverse Effects Affecting Patients after Discharge from the Hospital," Annals of Internal Medicine, 2003, 138: 161-7

363.  Boockvar, K, "Adverse Effects Due to Discontinuations in Drug Use and Dose Change in Patients Transferred Between Acute and Long Term Facilities," Archives of Internal Medicine, 2004, 164: 545-50

364. Steunser, D, "The Rise of Nursing home Litigation: Findings from a National Survey of Attorneys," Health Affairs, 2003, 22(2): 219-29

365. Kapp, M, "Nursing Home Culture Change: Legal Apprehensions and Opportunities," The Gerontologist, 2013, 53(5): 718-26

366. Gozalo, "End of Life Transitions among Nursing Home Residents with Cognitive Issues," New England Journal of Medicine, 2011, 365: 1212-20

367. Fried, T, "Fragility and Hospitalization of Long Term Stay Nursing Home Residents," Journal of the American Geriatric Society, 1997, 45(3): 265-9

368. Barker, W, "Rates, Patterns, Causes, and Costs of Hospitalization of Nursing Home Residents: A Population Based Study," American Journal of Public Health, 1994, 84(10): 165-20

369. Intrator, O, "Facility Characteristics Associated with Hospitalization of Nursing Home Residents: Results of a National Study," Medical Care, 1999, 37(3): 228-37

370. Byock, The Best Care Possible, pg. 45.

371. Grunier, A, "Hospitalization of Nursing Home Residents with Cognitive Impairments: The Influence of Organizational Features and State Policies," Gerontologist, 2007, 47: 447-56

372. Byock, The Best Care Possible, pp. 103, 112.

373. www.medpac.gov/chapter/mar12_ch11.pdf, pg. 284

374. www.nytimes.com\2011\6\28\health

375. Whoriskey, P, "In Hospice, but not Dying," The Washington Post, December 27, 2013, pg. 1.

376. "Nursing Home or Hospital: The Medical Director's Response to Increasing Medical Acuity," AMDA Long Term Care Conference, 3/21-24, 2013.

377. Prasad, V, "President Bush's Unnecessary Surgery," The Washington Post, pg. A23.

378. Fernandez, E, "Aggressive Surgery for Nonfatal Skin Cancers Might Not be Best for all Elderly Patients," April 29, 2013,

www.ucsf.edu/news/2013/04/105436/surgery-nonfatal-skin-cancers-might-not-be-best-elderly-patients.

379.   Rosenthal, E, "Patients' Costs Skyrocket; Specialists' Incomes Soar," The New York Times, January 18, 2014

380.        www.forbes.com/sites/markhendrickson/2013/03/07/did-you-really-pay-for-your-medicare-benefits/

381.   Brownlee, Overtreated, pp. 269-87

382.   Meisel, Z, "Post-HOM Health Care: Are ACO's the answer?" Time, www.time.com/time/health/article/0.8599.2074816.00

383.   Abramson, Overdosed America, pg. 81

384.   Angus, DC, "The Effect of Managed Care on ICU Length of Stay: Implications for Medicare," JAMA, 1996, 276: 1075-82

385.   Boodman, S, "The 1% Solution," The Washington Post, October 18, 2013, pg. E1.

386.   www.innovations.cms.gov

387.   www.hhs.gov/opa/affordable-care-act/index.html

388.   Zamosky, L, "Will a New Anti-fraud Campaign Lead to More Audits?" Medical Economics, October 25, 2013

389.   www.physicianspractice.com/blog/six-main-reasons-physicians-are-dropping-medicare-patients

390.   "Do Electronic Medical Records Save Money?" The New York Times, editorial, March 6, 2012

391.   Kliff, S, "Why Electronic Health Records Failed," The Washington Post, January 11, 2013

392.   Japsen, B, "Half of US Patients can Access Obamacare's 'Accountable Care Organizations,'" Forbes, www.forbes.com/sites/brusejapsen/2013/02/18

393.   Northern Maryland Collaborative Care, Provider Handbook, www.northermdcc.com

394.   AMDA Long Term Care Conference, 3/21-3/24, 2013: Adams, D "ACO's: Payer Driven Innovations in LTC," and Nichols, J, "What a Medical Director Needs to Know about Bundled Payment's and ACO's."

395.   Rau, J, "Medicare Speeds up Pay Plan," <u>Washington Post</u>, July 22, 2013, pg. A15.

396.   www.northernmdcc.com. Provider Handbook.

397.   Doughler, N, "Can Accountable Care organizations Improve Population Health?" <u>JAMA</u>, 2013, 309(111), pg. 119

398.   Landon, B, "Keeping Score Under a Global Payment System," <u>New England Journal of Medicine</u>, 2012, 366: 393-5

399.   Rittenhouse, D, "Primary Care and Accountable Care—Two essential Elements of Delivery-system-reform," <u>New England Journal of Medicine</u>, 2009, 361: 2301-3

400.   Burns, L, "Accountable Care Organizations may have Difficulty Avoiding the Failures of Integrative Delivery Networks of the 1990's," <u>Health Affairs</u>, 2012, 31(11): 2407-16

401.   www.En-wikipedia.org/wiki/diagnosis-related-group

402.   Ezekiel, J, "Saving by the Bundle," <u>The New York Times</u>, November 16, 2011

403.   Weeks, W, "The Unintended Consequences of Bundled Payments," <u>Annals of Internal Medicine</u>, 2013, 158(1): 62-4

404.   Naylor, M, "Unintended Consequences of Steps to Cut Readmissions and Reform Payment may Threaten Care of Vulnerable Older Adults," <u>Health Affairs</u>, 2012, 31(7): 1023-36

405.   Nichols, J, "What a Medical Director Needs to Know About Bundled Payments and ACO's," AMDA Long Term Conference, 2013.

406.   Jaspen, B, "Through Obamacare Pays Less, Providers Flock to 'Bundled' Medicare Payments," <u>Forbes</u>, February 1, 2013

407.   Flood, K, "Effect of an Acute Care for Elders Unit on costs and Thirty Day Readmissions," <u>JAMA</u>, 2013, 173(11): 981-7

408.   www.aamc.org/advocacy/medicare/153896/independent-payment-advisory-board-ipab.html

409.   Dean, H, "The ACA's Rate Setting Won't Work," <u>The Wall Street Journal</u>, July 28, 2013.

410.   www.thehealtcareblog.com/blog/tag/peter-orszag/

411.   Vestal, C, "Maryland may be the Model for Curbing Hospital Costs," USA Today, January 31, 2014. http://www.usatoday.com/story/news/nation/2014/01/31/stateline-maryland-hospital-costs/5079073

412.   Loggers, E, "Implementing a Death with Dignity Program at a Comprehensive Cancer Center," New England Journal of Medicine, 2013, 368(15): 1417-24

413.   Byock, Ira, The Best Care Possible, Avery, NY, 2012

414.   Jaffe, S, "Report Faults Care at Nursing Homes," The Washington Post, March 7, 2014, P. A16.

415.   Emanuel, E, "Shorten Medical Training by 30%," JAMA, 2012, 307(11): 1043-44.

416.   Boodman, S, "Fast Track Through Medical School," The Washington Post, January 14, 2014, pg. E1.

417.   www.medicare.gov

418.   Verghese, J, "Leisure Activities and the Risk of Dementia in the Elderly," New England Journal of Medicine, 2003, 348: 2508-16

417.   Gregg, EW, "Relationship of Changes in Physical Activity and Mortality among Older Women," New England Journal of Medicine, 2003, 289(8): 2379-86

420.   Lautenschlage, "Effect of Physical Activity on Cognitive Function in Older Adults at Risk of Alzheimer's Disease," JAMA, 2008, 300: 1027-37

421.   Larson, "Exercise is Associated with Reduced Risk of Dementia in the Elderly," New England Journal of Medicine, 2003, 348: 2508-11